The Celtic Holy Grail Quest

By David Stocks

'One million people commit suicide every year.'
The World Health Organization

David Stocks

All rights reserved, no part of this publication may be reproduced by any means, electronic, mechanical photocopying, documentary, film or in any other format without prior written permission of the publisher.

Published by
Chipmunkapublishing
PO Box 6872
Brentwood
Essex CM13 1ZT
United Kingdom
http://www.chipmunkapublishing.com

Copyright © David Stocks 2008

Edited by Linda Zamboglou

The Celtic Holy Grail Quest

Dedication

I dedicate this book to Jules, my soul mate and Lady in waiting, without whom this book would never have been possible.

David Stocks

The Celtic Holy Grail Quest

Chapter 1 Interference on the radio

The interior of the office was modern, but alone there at night the atmosphere of the old chapel it had once been was freed to creep into my bones. Despite the heating, a chill seemed to pervade the building. It was as if the structure was reverting back to a place of solitude and worship, a house of spirits. Spirits, whose cold fingers crept up my spine and seeped into my mind, reaching into those hidden places where the night demons dwell and stirring the depths within. My fingers were stiff and cold, as they clicked their way across the keyboard. I believed I could smell the mustiness of accumulated time. My concentration wavered. I listened to the unheard whispers which reverberated around the room. On screen the grid of database links became random and un-sequenced. I tried to fit them back together by clicking on a dead data source.

Like a dead data source? Like the dead that laid buried beneath the floor of this chapel of modern usage. A stream of binary digits pervaded the screen, even before I was able to connect it to a database. The glow of the marching digits (1101000101001001) dazzled my eyes. The secret murmurs grew louder as these digits spewed forth in an electronic whisper. Were they echoing the silent voices of the dead?

Out of the highly organised computer structures on which I was working, chaos was being

David Stocks

generated. In a world of logic, randomness was prevailing. This place was playing with my head. Time to go home! I printed a screen dump for later analysis, shut down my computer and switched off the lights. The pools of ghostly moonlight fell across the room, shining in through the Gothic arched windows and casting furtive shadows into the inner recesses of the room.

Deep in the corner I saw the dark outline of a cowled monk standing watching me from the shadows. Fear embraced me in its freezing hold, splinters of ice passed through my body and down my spine. Tiny follicles of hair stood on end all over my tautened skin that bristled with static energy. My heart momentarily stopped, as I stood cast like a wax figurine in a dungeon of horrors, awaiting my unknown fate at the hands of ancient supernatural forces.
My vision reeled in the darkness; black images swam in the unholy moonlight, indistinct, unclear, brooding and dangerous. I was trapped in this forlorn chapel, the way to the door blocked by the spectral monk. Slowly my eyes adjusted to their dark surroundings, outlines of objects took on more form as I tuned in to the dim light in much the same way a TV tunes in to a channel; white noise, static, slowly resolving into distinct images. Seconds passed as eons in my petrified state, dark imaginings of my mind taking on their most fearful forms. My rational conscious thought processes were lost in a storm of primitive fears, buried deep in the subconscious. What manner of

The Celtic Holy Grail Quest

spirit now walked this place? What fate awaited me this lonely night?

I tensed as my fight or flight instincts kicked in. I was not religious but I prayed for God's help all the same. At the point of action, my vision finally cleared and there before me stood not a ghoulish monk, but my coat hanging by its hood from the coat stand. Darkness and my weary state had been playing tricks on my mind.
I retrieved the monk, put on my coat and pulled up my hood. Now, monk-like myself I headed into the night. I felt like a modern disciple born into the religion of technology, a follower of secret network links and hidden databases of dark knowledge, a worshiper of the God of the internet and the World Wide Web. A fleeting thought passed through my mind. Had a God encouraged man to create the internet and, if so, what better way to distribute knowledge and wisdom? Or is it the devil's work; a dark spider waiting for unsuspecting prey on its electronically spun World Wide Web? The battle for good and evil is waged on many levels. Are technology and the internet the latest battleground?

With these musings in mind, I set off on the long road from Leamington Spa to Nottingham, eager to return to the warmth and companionship of my wife and home. I switched on the radio. As I travelled fog began to swirl into the crisp clear night. The stars misted up and the fog unrolled its carpet along the road. The radio lost reception and

David Stocks

its friendly voice died back to a quiet background hiss. Blindly I followed the car in front, its red tail lights burning through the fog like angry red eyes. The creepy atmosphere was getting to me. Was something sinister watching me, waiting for me to make a mistake?

The journey was interminable - I lost track of speed and time. I followed my ghostly leader on our midnight journey through the nothingness of the fog bank. My mind wandered and my body went onto autopilot. A motorbike came the other way, its headlight throwing out our images into the fog, like a projector onto a swirling silver screen. I was a movie star, part of a celluloid fantasy; techno kid, drifting through cyberspace, following an internet daemon down to its lair.

Disorientated and lost, I was travelling I knew not where. I lived to follow my satanic leader. Was this wise? I was lost without bearings, compulsively following someone or something. My eyes grew heavy and the mist dragged me further down after it. As it was about to totally engulf my consciousness, the sound of my name called from the depths of the radio static jogged me awake.

'Dave … Dave,' it said. Startled, I swerved and almost careered off the road. Through the crackle and hiss something had called my name. Whatever it was had saved my life. Alert again I focussed on what little I could see of the road. The car in front of me was gone. I passed a sign on the

The Celtic Holy Grail Quest

roadside, 'Wolvey.' Weariness washed over me. I pulled up by the entrance to a field, reclined the car seat and quickly gave in to drowsiness.

I drifted off to the realms of the unconscious and was surrounded by dark androgynous figures, with deep furnace-like eyes, burning bright as the car lights I had so recently been following. They moved around me in a swirling dance, gyrating and spinning, appearing and disappearing, moving in and out of focus, never static, always indiscernible. In the background I could hear a rhythmic beat, not like drums, something more hollow and wooden. It was resonating and emanating from deep within the earth. The dancing became faster and with it the rhythm intensified. I felt a primitive force as old as time, an ancient terrestrial power. Mother Earth was speaking and I was being dragged down into her earthen folds, becoming one with the planet. Engulfed in a geological blanket, I tasted the metallic essence of terra firma on my tongue and was soon overwhelmed. Choking, I awoke with a start, disorientated and sick with the aftertaste of soil in my mouth.

The fog had lifted and now a large full moon hung above the horizon, casting a baleful yellow glow on the road ahead of me. It was surrounded by a ghostly halo. The road was a lunar highway heading directly towards this grim portent. The night resumed its creepy, surreal feel. The moon mesmerized me; it looked so big, a giant satellite orbiting the earth. It wasn't just a lump of rock, but an intelligent spy satellite on earth surveillance duty, put there by a cosmic being for an unknown purpose. It was watching me, but it wasn't friendly, it was distinctly malevolent.

I was in a monochromatic, sepia-tinted world, a place of dark shadows and demons, a world devoid of colour; a lonely and frightening zone where evil spirits dwelled. I felt both agoraphobic and claustrophobic at the same time. The vast expanse of the universe was spread out before me. I was a microscopic dot in an infinitesimal field of giant stars. I was so minute, the scale of the universe so vast, that I felt totally worthless, yet at the same time I felt hemmed in and sensed I was being watched. I couldn't escape; I was enclosed in a prison cell with its walls pushing in towards me. I was entering an unfamiliar world I didn't like and couldn't understand. All my energy was drained and I could feel only despair and despondency. I had crossed a line drawn across my mind and I had no map to find my way back.

I drove on, keen to reach home and normality. I was on the Old Fosse, an ancient roman road, which now carried my modern steel chariot. As I travelled the roads of ancient Britain I perceived a raw primeval power which the modern world fails to understand. I was trapped in a time capsule with no option but to journey to its ultimate destination. The road was rough and uneven beneath my wheels, like the cobbled roads of

The Celtic Holy Grail Quest

Roman times. Trees lined its sides, like Roman sentinels protecting my passage against the marauding hordes of Britons. The huge feverish yellow globe of the moon hovered over this lunar highway, beckoning me on along its sinister path. I put my foot down; I needed to leave this ancient track as soon as possible. The trees closed in on me from all sides, forcing me to drive faster to escape their gnarled grasp. All around was a thickening forest, backlit by the ghostly moonlight, branches like black sinuous arms clawing at the heavens. Why had I never noticed so many trees, why had I not seen this forest before?

It was with much relief that I eventually reached the turn-off to Nottingham. I swept off the Old Fosse without slowing. The moon still kept a vigilant watch over me, but I felt a release of tension as I left the Fosse behind me.

The remaining miles passed in a blur. I remember arriving home to the old village centre of Gamston. Gamston has grown vastly since I first moved there, but its centre remains old. On the tiny, triangular-shaped village green stands a wooden village hall. This ancient green was lit up by the moonlight and I felt the weight of millennia pressing onto it, but no way was I going to explore it that night.

My cottage was in a courtyard, just across from the green and more tension eased from my shoulders as I pulled up. My wife was already

David Stocks

asleep and so I went straight to bed, but sleep wasn't easy coming. My mind was a whirl of thoughts and images. I lay in a semiconscious stupor, the yellow moonlight twitching at the curtains. Even the quiet breathing of my wife couldn't drive out my fear. Still I was being watched! In my anxiety I hid under the duvet, but I didn't know from what I was hiding. My skin was cold and clammy. A deep fear was growing in my mind nurturing the seeds of self-doubt.

The Celtic Holy Grail Quest

Chapter 2 Closed mind stasis, lunar dream cycle

I awoke the next morning, or did I? I was neither awake nor asleep, disconnected from reality, but denied the ultimate escape of sleep. I lay restless, disengaged from the regular world, anxiety sweeping over me like a wave. I was drowning in my worries; my bed had become a life raft that I clung on to. If I just stayed there, in my bed, I wouldn't have to face the rest of the world. I wouldn't have to confront that endless journey to and from work. No need to touch a computer, weave logic patterns across a screen, whilst analysing a crash dump on another screen. I couldn't face work that day, even if I could get up! I felt like all the energy had been siphoned from me like a spent battery. I phoned in sick; I had a virus I told them. This was in fact partly true; I had been infected by a virus, a computer virus! Computers had taken over my life, their binary patterns had imprinted themselves on my brain and now my body wanted to reject it. I no longer wanted to be part of their world of cold logic, ingesting and regurgitating data, to satisfy the corporate thirst for information processing.

In my mind I enclosed my brain within a spherical shield; a chromium-plated mirrored surface providing protection from all digital influence. Safe from penetration by the ever pervading digital pollution that forms electronic smog in our modern world of satellites, cellular phones and high speed network communications. The digital hiss reflected back by my mind's defences and all existing data expelled from my body, exuded from my pores, bit by binary bit. Safe behind my mental shield, I withdrew from reality and entered a state of cerebral stasis.

I visited the doctor and was given medication to help combat stress. He also signed me off work for a couple of weeks. The pills didn't have any noticeable effect, my mood continued to dip and I could no longer sleep. The medication was increased and sleeping tablets were added to my ever increasing pharmaceutical cocktail. With this addition I finally managed to sleep, but not a restful sleep, rather a tortured nocturnal journey of fevered dreams, which gave me no refreshment in body or spirit afterwards. I dreamt of trees, huge oak trees all around me. I ran through a forest and the trees were reaching out their gnarled branches, trying to grasp me. I felt trapped, nowhere to go, with the moon watching me from above, casting its sickly yellow light down upon the forest. In front of me appeared a horned figure silhouetted against the moon, like some mythical beast from old. With a shiver I awoke, snapping my eyes open, a cold sweat on my body.

I had many variations of this dream, the worst being set in a forest, but instead of trees I found myself in amongst a thicket of electricity pylons. The pylons were all around me and I was trying to

The Celtic Holy Grail Quest

find a path through them. It was twilight and the sky was a deep blue. The moon hung on the horizon, a silver disc infusing the sky with an electric hue. Pulses of electrical current sped along the power lines above me. A strong smell of ozone hung in the air and I had a sharp metallic taste in my mouth. I was enveloped in a field of static electricity, the hairs on my body vibrated, prickling my skin with their static charge. Under a darkening sky, clouds swept across the moon. Above me the power lines hummed, still discharging blue sparks of electricity. The whole atmosphere thickened into an electrical soup, as the heavens brought their own fusion of electricity to play in the form of a dark thunderstorm. Lightening struck down from the skies, smashing into the pylons, which in turn sent electricity shooting back up into the atmosphere. The noise was deafening as the air was wrenched apart from above and below, seemingly tearing the fabric of reality asunder, columns of pure blue energy arced throughout the ionosphere. A concussive shock wave threw me to the ground and I lay face up to the sky.

Pillars of raw power formed between the pylons and the sky, dispersing their energy in great electrical waves across the bottom of the clouds. The undulations of the clouds resembled the contours and folds of a gargantuan brain. Electric pulses shot between its synapses, an elemental brain governing the forces of nature, an environmental entity. Could nature actually be a conscious, thinking process, all part of a global mind? As this idea formed, the storm began to disperse and through a gap in the clouds I could see the moon. It hung there full and clear, silhouetted against it stood the twisted wreckage of an electricity pylon, looking eerily like a horned figure. Ancient myth turned modern? The pylon then began to topple towards me, power cables whipping loose and snapping out at me like the tentacles of an angry sea monster, sparking and dancing within inches of my stunned body. I awoke with a start, just as the pylon came crashing down on me. Every hair on my body stood on end, as if I had been in the presence of a massive amount of electricity. My whole body shuddered and twitched as the current drained from within, leaving me limp and perspiring on the bed, all my body's electrical energy spent in vividly active dreams.

My mind, which had become insular and dormant when awake, was now highly active and energetic when asleep. Subconsciously I was functioning, but my conscious state was not responding at all. I needed to somehow reverse the polarity, so that my consciousness became active and subconscious turned more quiescent. I needed to rewire my body, but how? The brain's circuitry is a highly complex organic computer, driven by millions of electrochemical impulses, with a wiring diagram that is virtually impossible to understand. Once a fault develops in the software that runs on this computer, it is very difficult to rectify;

The Celtic Holy Grail Quest

debugging it was going to be difficult and I didn't know where to start?

The answer came to me when I started seeing a therapist. By this time I was off long term sick and he encouraged me to involve myself in something, get an activity, and engage the mind. This advice is very sound, but to someone in a highly depressed state it is very hard to break free from the overwhelming lethargic despondency that is present inside. It took much coaxing and encouragement from doctors, my wife and family, but with their help and an inner determination I applied myself to exercising my mind. Using my dreams as a starting point, I became fascinated as to whether they had any meaning or source and undertook research into understanding my dreams, to query the fundamental mechanisms of my subconscious, to find the origin of my dreams and equip myself with the tools to tackle my anxiety.

A stone was cast into the pool of my mind; the ripples that emerged in all directions became the start of my quest for the Celtic Holy Grail. I did not know this at the time, but it was at this point my quest started and little did I know it was going to take me six years to complete it.

Chapter 3 Dreams and visions on the Old Fosse

I initiated my research with the first dream I'd had at Wolvey on the Old Fosse.

I trawled the local libraries in search of material I could use to interpret my nocturnal travels. Armed with an admirable haul of books and documents, I returned home to study them and begin my dream interpretation.

My first point of reference was a map of old Roman roads. On this the Old Fosse was clearly marked and Wolvey stood at the intersection of the Fosse and another old Roman road. This junction was marked on the map as High Cross. Further research unravelled the history of the road and its primeval origins. Prior to the Roman construction of the road, it had already been used as an early pathway for 2000 years. Significantly, arial studies of High Cross still show the traces of a truly ancient Henge monument that had once stood at this juncture.

Could this be a meeting place where sacred rituals were once performed? I could almost feel Britain's Celtic past calling me as I immersed myself further into my research. I had embarked on an ancient track, one that would take mind, body and spirit on a journey through long forgotten paths - of torment, loneliness and amnesia to awakening,

The Celtic Holy Grail Quest

friendship and enlightenment - a journey that would bring me face to face with the conflicts imposed by the modern world on our ancient planet.

Perhaps the dream I experienced at High Cross was a spiritual echo of rituals held there in the past? Celtic shamans may have used bodhrans (frame drums) to produce a hypnotic beat, whose rhythm their spirits danced to, inducing a trance-like state. From within this state they were able to commune with the spirits, asking for their help and guidance. Such a ceremony reflected my vivid encounter in the realm of dreams, dark conjurations dancing to another worldly beat.

During the course of my research on the horned figure haunting my dreams, I stumbled upon a Celtic god, 'Cernunnos,' Lord of the Beasts and giver of prosperity. He can also be seen in the guise of the 'Lord of the Hunt' who uses his shamanic powers to guide hunters on their quest for prey. This latter interpretation was to have a profound effect on me later, but now I remained blissfully ignorant.

It became ever more evident that my dreams were firmly rooted in our Celtic past, Celtic spirits calling me across eons, down to their mystical world of nature and forgotten realms, the real and surreal. I put my first tentative steps into the land of the Celts, searching their wisdom for help in overcoming my depression. I trawled through books, archives and maps, becoming engrossed in my work. Hefty volumes and tomes formed haphazard towers around me, threatening to collapse and engulf me in their ancient texts. After long journeys through Celtic literature I encountered references to the Holy Grail, this legend is steeped in Celtic mystery and it has its roots firmly embedded in Celtic Mythology.

I also referenced the meaning of dreams containing entangled power lines. Dreams of this kind are supposed to indicate a struggle for empowerment, be this in a relationship, at work, or achieving life's goals. The latter interpretation would seem to be the most apt, for deep inside me was a feeling of inadequacy, a feeling that I had an inner purpose that I was at that moment blind to, a purpose that became ever more clear to me as I undertook the path that led to the writing of this book.

I now had a purpose, I had a mission, I had awoken from a dream and been carried back on the mists of time, to the ancient land of the Celts. I must cast off the shackles of modernity and equip myself for the ultimate quest, harking back to the Legends of King Arthur and the Knights of the Round Table and still further back to its Celtic origins and the founding of the Grail legend. I was about to embark on a quest that would change my life, none other than the quest for the Holy Grail. Not from the usual starting point, in the tradition of the latter day Christian quest for Christ's Holy

The Celtic Holy Grail Quest

Chalice, but from the roots of the grail legend as a Celtic Knight seeking I'm not sure what?

Still fascinated by the site of my original dream I looked closely at this ancient Roman intersection of roads, marked High Cross. Untangling the threads that make up this Celtic knot I found a possible Celtic history of great significance to Britain. For High Cross marks the juncture of the old Roman roads of the Fosse and Watling Street. For those who know their British history, the battle of Watling Street was the battle in which the great British and Celtic Warrior Queen Boudicca was defeated in 60 or 61 AD. The site of this momentous battle is much disputed but one of the candidate locations is High Cross; the basis being that the Roman commander at the time retreated down Watling Street and united with reinforcements arriving from the Fosse. In the tradition of Boudicca, I fight invasion into my own protected realm of the mind, seeking to drive out my demons and in the process grasp what cannot be sought, the Holy Grail.

Chapter 4 Refugee from Hell

My Grail quest got off to a slow start, however, for my low mood continued to get the better of me until I found every waking moment a nightmare. The nightmare didn't cease with sleep, feverish dreams took me down to the sulphurous depths of hell, the place where my inner demons dwell.

I could no longer cope with the world and I cast myself adrift in a little boat called despair and was immediately swept out into a stormy sea of emotions. I nearly drowned in my own sorrow, while a raging tempest crashed against the walls of my mind and eventually washed me ashore on the beach of hopelessness, where I was taken in to the care of Queens Medical Centre hospital. This was the last bastion against my mind and it was there that I recovered from my torment, a refugee from hell.

My days in this island of calm, far from the fearful demons that were pursuing me, passed in a haze. My mind was no longer my own, numbed by the intensity of the emotions that had engulfed me, awash in a sea of medication. I was no longer aware of myself, or anything around me. I had become more of an automaton; I looked like a human being from the outside, but all I did was act out the role and no longer functioned on the cognitive level.

The Celtic Holy Grail Quest

Gaggles of doctors and psychiatrists would peer at me from behind facades of faces contorted by manic grins that are the trademark of their profession and ask me questions that I couldn't answer and didn't want to answer. I could reconcile with the so called heretics that were brought before the Spanish inquisition. I was paraded before an assortment of specialists and their student followers, who practised in the blind faith of their profession. As greater quantities and mixtures of drugs were deposited into my system I began to realise that mental health treatment was more of a black art than a science. Practitioners of this black art would huddle together and discuss my treatment, noting my reaction to the array of drugs in the shell of my body that had now become a human laboratory. I was oblivious to their machinations, remaining in a state of 'hell shock,' only time would heal the scars on my mind.

Weeks passed and my toxic tolerance to the substances I was imbibing increased and I surfaced from a stupor, slowly functioning again. I went to relaxation classes and managed to find a tranquil oasis in which to recuperate from my inner journey across the scorched desert of my consciousness.

This, coupled with the loving support of my wife and family, pulled me through my desperate times. Without this place of surrender I would never have made it; I thank my wife, family and all the staff at

David Stocks

the Queens Medical centre for getting me through those times. The doctors may have been practising scientific Voodoo, sticking hypodermic pins in me, but they did rescue me from the fiery pit of hell.

It was a changed person that left the hospital some weeks later, no longer a refugee, but forever baring the scars from my time in Dante's inferno.

The Celtic Holy Grail Quest

Chapter 5 Vision in the rain

Having extricated myself from the clutches of despair, with hell's dark shadow still shrouding me in its inky blackness, I took to continuing my Grail quest with vigour. The Grail quest was well documented, but its origins in Celtic legend was more difficult to uncover, with many twists and turns to catch out the unsuspecting.

References to the Grail within Celtic folklore were hard to pin down and difficult to unravel, so I decided to look farther afield to see if I could find anything more substantial. With this in mind, I set out with my wife for an antique bookshop in Lincoln, coincidentally along another stretch of the Old Fosse.

The air was heavy with precipitation, the sky overcast and murky. Everything was grimy, grey and uninviting. My spirit was deflated, my quest for information insignificant. Why should I bother? I felt detached from reality, my whole life now grey, swallowing me up in its ordinariness and regurgitating me back into drab urbanity. Nevertheless I carried on to Lincoln, simply because I didn't have the energy to turn back.

Gradually in the rain sodden gloom of the road ahead, a cyclist materialised on the opposite carriageway, moving imperceptibly towards me. He appeared to move slowly, but this was deceptive for despite the effortless way in which he cycled, the distance between us closed dramatically and I could soon make out his features. He was a tall, black man in a black suit, wearing a black overcoat open to the elements. I say he was black, but he was not black as in the colour, he was more an absence of colour. He didn't reflect light back at all; light just fell into him, disappearing into a dark void. He peddled calmly on, as if he owned the road and there was nobody else on it. As this black rider peddled past me, I felt time slip and run backwards. I checked for him in my mirror, but he was no longer there, lost in the rain and the ever-spinning wheels of time. I commented to my wife that I had seen him, but she looked bemused and said she had seen no cyclist at all.

I felt that I had just experienced a waking dream. My conscious and subconscious worlds were crossing over, the lines of distinction between the two blurring. I had entered the mysterious world of lucid dreaming, this being the most presentable option to me, other options of spirits past and present or dark unknown forces I did not even want to contemplate.

The rest of the journey passed without incident. As we approached Lincoln I could see the Cathedral standing prominently on top of a hill. Its mighty form was standing stark, like a dark citadel against the brooding storm clouds above it. Lincoln has a castle, but it is the Cathedral that dominates the

The Celtic Holy Grail Quest

landscape.

Parking near the Cathedral we walked inside and saw the famous Lincoln Imp on a pillar above us. There was something in the way it peered down on me with a malevolent grin that made me cold inside. I could feel its evil stare pervading the inner sanctum of my body, searching for my most guarded internal fears. I stood rooted to the spot unable to move, yet wanting to flee. My wife tugged on my arm and pulled me away from the spot. I felt the cold grasp of fear tug on my soul as I was jerked away. The imp had made its indelible mark on me, an unseen attachment, the shackles of which would impede me every step of the way upon my Grail quest. I tried to shake off the ill feeling that engulfed my being and admire the majesty of the place. The scale of the cathedral was astonishing, the grandeur of its vaulted ceilings, the majesty of its gothic windows and the weightlessness of its flying buttresses was breathtaking. But what purpose did an evil imp serve, lurking high up in the shadows within the house of God?

Afterwards we made our way down the aptly named 'Steep Hill.' The rain was torrential and it cascaded down the hill, making it very difficult to keep our footing, especially on the cobbled surface. We had to cling on to each other tightly to avoid sliding on the flood of water streaming down the hill and ending up like discarded driftwood, flotsam and jetsam, seemingly hurled from the lofty reaches of Lincoln's old town. Not surprisingly we were the only people foolhardy enough to venture onto Steep Hill in those conditions and it was with some surprise that the antique bookshop owner greeted us when we stumbled, wet and bedraggled into his lonely temple of the written word.

The shopkeeper was an old man, but not stooped and haggard, rather he was dignified and timeworn. He was comfortably dressed in tweed trousers and a chequered shirt, over which he wore a black waistcoat embroidered with golden sundial motifs. His face was welcoming, with its warm tanned skin, textured but not creased with age. His eyes were intense, but at the same time friendly. It amazed me how people take on the physical characteristics of their occupation. He appeared to me as an old leather tome, inviting me to open the cover and soak up the information within.

'Any port in a storm is it?' he asked.
'No, I have in fact come specifically to visit your renowned shop,' I replied.
'I am honoured,' he said. 'So what can I do for you?'

I explained that I was after some information on Celtic myths, particularly ones associated with the Grail legend.

'Ah, Celtic myths, the Grail legend? You may find

The Celtic Holy Grail Quest

what you are looking for hard to find!' the shopkeeper said. 'The trouble with Celtic history is that they didn't write anything down. All their knowledge, history, religion, myths and legends were passed on orally through Bardic verses. Some of these took as long as twenty years to learn. Later texts on the Celts were written by the Romans and Monks, but these could well have been distorted from the original by Christian writers and their prejudices.'

I felt dejected, to have journeyed so far through relentless rain for nothing.

Looking at my downcast expression he smiled, 'I can point you in the right direction, though. I am actually a Celtic scholar and have had the fortune to speak to one of the few remaining people who has carried on the Bardic tradition. He is simply known as Old Tom and lives in Ireland. Ireland and Wales have the most complete Celtic history. He is one of the last shanachie, or storytellers, and is essentially a keeper of Celtic wisdom. He says that the Celtic way of life is one that is in harmony with Mother Nature and if you find this harmony inner peace will follow. The Holy Grail - you do right to look for the Holy Grail in Celtic Mythology. Most Grail seekers are blinkered by modern writings of the Holy Grail and the Christian emphasis that it has been given as that of a cup containing the blood of Christ. True Grail seekers look beyond this adaptation of the Grail legend and further into its roots in the Celtic underworld.

David Stocks

The precise nature of the Grail is hard to pin down though; some say it is a cauldron imbued with magical properties of the underworld, including rejuvenation and wisdom, but there is a lot more to it than that. One thing I will say is that the Holy Grail is something that can only be found by following and understanding the Celtic way.'

Intrigued I left the shop clutching three volumes on Celtic lore to aid me in unravelling the mysteries and beliefs of the Celtic way of life. I also left uplifted, for the shopkeeper radiated good feeling and I felt I had found a friend there. At that moment friends were what I needed most. He also left me his card and said if ever I needed any help then I must not hesitate in contacting him. I took his card, accepting it not as a business card, but as a token of friendship.

The Celtic Holy Grail Quest

Chapter 6 Grail Lore, following the Celtic way: The true quest begins

A prolonged period of study into Grail lore and the origins of the Holy Grail legend pursued. There are many interpretations of the Holy Grail legend and many possible sources for its Arthurian characters, quest and ultimately the Grail itself. It is impossible to pinpoint any one true source for the story; it rather seems an amalgamation of many different tales and myths. One common feature though, is the inspiration for the Holy Grail quest, which is very much of Celtic origin.

At the beginning of the first millennium B.C., Britain and Ireland were one of the last bastions of the Celtic people standing against the mighty Roman Empire, the remote Islands tucked away in a far corner of the globe surrounded by sea. It wasn't until the 7th century A.D. that Celtic Britain was finally vanquished, leaving behind only through its much diminished Celtic-speaking descendants, the Myths and Legends of the Celtic people, only fragments of which remain today.

The Christian church assimilated a great deal of the Celtic and ancient Briton Folklore into their Christian Dogma. These were incorporated in Medieval Christian Tales, amalgamating them into Christian beliefs and filling them with Christian Virtues of the Medieval period. The source of the modern day interpretation of the Holy Grail quest can very much be put down to the 13th Century

David Stocks

French writer Chrétien de Troyes in the 'Conte del Graal.' The origins of the word 'Grail' most likely go back to the Latin word 'Cratalis' meaning bowl. The association of the Grail being Christ's cup is pretty thin, especially with the abundant host of otherworld Celtic cauldrons in Celtic Mythology.

Early in the 13th century, Robert de Borron's poem Joseph d'Arimathie, or the Roman de l'estoire dou Graal, extended the Christian significance of the legend. Robert de Borron's poem recounted the Grail's early history, linking it with the cup used by Christ at the Last Supper and afterwards by Joseph of Arimathea to catch the blood flowing from Christ's wounds as he hung upon the Cross. This was later brought back to England by Joseph d'Arimathie. The Fisher King had received a terrible and un-healing wound to the groin, which had been pierced by the lance that had also gashed the side of Jesus' side on the cross. Because of his suffering the Kingdom was reduced to a desolate wasteland. Only the sacred power of the holy chalice entrusted to the Fisher King, the Holy Grail, sustained the King and Kingdom. Perceval, a knight of modest background and upbringing, took on the quest for the Holy Grail. On his first meeting with the Fisher King, he found the magical Grail Castle, but forgot to ask the question, 'Whom does the Grail Serve?' On his second meeting with the Fisher King, distraught and weakened by time and fate, he remembers to ask the question, 'Whom does the Grail serve?' The King replies, 'Those who serve

The Celtic Holy Grail Quest

the Grail.' At that moment the King and Kingdom are healed.

The first part of the Vulgate cycle, called 'Estoire del Saint Graal,' provides the most in-depth early history of the Grail. As well as discussing the origin of the Grail (a relic that touched Christ's lips and carried his blood, which was transported to Britain by Joseph of Arimathea), it gives an original account of Merlin, as a forest dwelling Druid with the gift of prophecy and magic. Here he is known as Celidone. This brings a likely comparison with Merlin Celidonius, a famous Welsh god. They both undergo mysterious death rites involving a tower as children; they both live a life in the woods and both study the stars and have a preternatural knowledge.

In an early Welsh poem, 'Preiddeu Annwyn' ('The spoils of Annwyn,') King Arthur sets sail for Annwn, the Celtic otherworld, or the Land of the Dead. It recounts a raid into this Celtic otherworld to steal 'The Cauldron of the Head of Annwn,' a powerful magical device. It is a disastrous mission, in which only seven of Arthur's warriors return. The Cauldron, being called 'The Head of Annwn,' has given rise to misconceptions. 'The Head' refers to the 'King of the Land' and 'Annwn' where the cauldron is located. The grail cannot be found by anyone who is not pure of spirit; the cauldron will not cook food for anyone who is a coward.

The origins of Merlin can be found in a sixth

century Welsh prince, Myrddin ab Morfyn appearing in a ninth century epic piece of Celtic literature Y Goddodin (The Goddodin), which recounts a fateful raid by a band of Celtic warriors (from a place close to the modern day Edinburgh) on a place known as Catraeth (close to the North Yorkshire town of Catterick). They fight a heavy battle against the Saxons, in which most are slain. Amongst those named is a Warrior called Myrdin (Merlin?), although nothing is told of his role or character.

A collection of poetic triplets dating back to the thirteenth century, Trioedd Ynys Prydein (The Triads of Britain), an aide-memoir for storytellers and poets, mentions Merlin. These preserve an oral tradition that dates a lot further back to the sixth century at least. 'Triad 87' lists:

> Three skilful bards of Arthur's Court:
> Myrddin son of Morfren,
> Myrddin Emrys,
> And Taliesin.

This is the first time that Merlin is associated with Arthur and it also suggests that there may have been more than one Merlin. The only possible link that can be found to Morfen is quite interesting. Morfran vab Tegid, who is also known as Agfaggdu ('Utter Darkness' or 'Great Cow') is the hideously ugly son of the goddess Ceridwen, for whom she brews a magical drink which will make him all-wise. The distillation of wisdom, known as

The Celtic Holy Grail Quest

'the three drops of inspiration,' is accidentally imbibed by a youth set to watch over Ceridwen's cauldron. He at once has access to all knowledge and after a chase in which he and the goddess shape-shift through several forms, the youth is reborn as Taliesin, the famous bard and shaman of sixth-century Britain, who is listed alongside Merlin in this triad.

Could this be the origins of the Holy Grail, with the character Merlin and a magic vessel (cauldron)?

There is much history of the Grail and also its Celtic roots that I have omitted here. If I were to list all the possible links making up the Celtic Holy Grail story in detail, you would be reading an immense book, full of interacting, transforming and sometimes conflicting information about the origins of the Grail and leaving you in an ever more confused state. I have not been able to clarify the exact nature of the Grail at this juncture, but I have resolved some key areas to look into.

And so a mighty tale is spun, from many different origins and beliefs. The difficulty I now have is unravelling the various threads of the legend and finding the true Grail hidden in amongst all of this history and mythology. From the insights I have gained into the nature of the Grail so far, I am going to align myself with the Celtic beliefs of living with nature and looking for openings into the otherworld (or underworld) where the Grail may exist.

David Stocks

Exploring the Celtic roots of the Grail further, the Grail is neither a cup or a Cauldron, but rather a magic vessel in which the dew of the otherworld gathered.

One piece of advice that I gleaned from the many books that I read, was to look for signs and follow your intuition. What signs these might be I didn't know, but I took the advice to heart and used it throughout the rest of this quest.

Little did I know at this stage, how many signs there would be and the many different directions that they would lead me. Like an intricate Celtic knot, I would follow the signs through their many twists and turns and follow the truths that were revealed at their mysterious intersections. Fellow Grail knight, follow me through the labyrinth of this book and don't forget to tread down unmarked paths by the wayside, for it is within these unknown regions that often the greatest secrets are to be found.

The Celtic Holy Grail Quest

Chapter 7 Insidious whispering

Following my trip to Lincoln, the disagreeable atmosphere I had felt in the cathedral persisted upon my return home. Bleak, cheerless days ensued; a damp chill crept into my bones draining me of what little energy I had. I descended into lethargy and melancholy. In this state I began to fall prey to voices, from where I knew not.

At first it was just a faint hiss, like a vent of steam seeping into my ears, gradually to become whispers. It was like I had demons sat on each shoulder whispering to each other through my ears. I played host to a demonic conversation, ridiculing me. They had found a soul who was weak in mind and spirit, an imperfect individual on which to practise their infernal ways. Their conversations washed through my brain, from ear to ear like waves, which sometimes crashed together in the middle, sending up plumes of expletives to all regions of my brain. Whispering taunts and feeding on my despair, they began to drown me in self loathing, despondency and sorrow. Their goal was for me to take my own life and send me to eternal damnation. They spoke as follows:

'He hath ears of the dead for he can hear us.'
'Such a worthless man as I have ever seen.'
'Despair not, for despair has already engulfed him.'

David Stocks

'Cannot he see the hopelessness of life?'
'He has no faith, there is no faith, for faith will not save him.'
'He walks the path of the dead, but even in death there is no salvation.'
'Never did such a miserable life exist. Die and do us all a favour.'

These voices drove me to a new level of despondency and it was in an effort to escape their clutches that I vowed to continue my research. I started reading a book that I had bought from Lincoln on the history of the cathedral.

Skimming through its contents I came across a chapter that intrigued me about the Lincoln Imp. The story told about the imp is that it was one of two wicked imps that were sent by Satan to perform his diabolical work. They initially created mischief by sitting on Chesterfield's spire and twisting it out of shape until it became crooked. After this they visited Lincoln and created havoc by tripping up the bishop and smashing tables and chairs. It was when they were trying to destroy the cathedral's angel choir that an angel intervened, telling them to stop at once. One of the imps fled, but the other braver fellow flew up to sit on a pillar. As punishment it was turned to stone and now sits on the pillar forever.

This myth reminded me of the little demons that I believed were sitting on my shoulders. Was it

The Celtic Holy Grail Quest

possible that during my visit to Lincoln Cathedral, the evil spirit of these diabolical little imps had taken up residence on my shoulders and deep inside my mind? I could picture them in my mind's eye about eight inches high, squat creatures with horns, batwing ears, wide sneering mouths and dragon-like tails, wearing ancient tunics; the very image of the devil's fiendish servants. Somehow I had to block them out of my mind, to which they had full access and were now playing on my deepest darkest fears and relaying them back to me. I now knew who I was facing, but how was I going to stop them? The battlefield was my mind, the prize was my soul.

Logic and doctors said of these troublesome voices, that they were just a creation of my mind, susceptible to devious subconscious machinations, in the weary and exhausted state it was currently in. To one whose thoughts had turned to darkness, they were the devil's own demons, there to guide me down to the fiery pits of hell.

By this time of my illness extreme lethargy had set in and the more I gave in to it, the greater was my weariness. To combat this I took to exercising and became a frequent visitor to the gym. The hardest thing was raising the energy to go to the gym, as I was so tired that I could not imagine doing anything physical. However, when I did, I soon found that exhaustion ebbed away and exercise actually filled me with positive energy. What's more, physical activity helped to keep the imps away and give my mind a rest from their constant mental assault.

After exercise I always felt good for a while, but this didn't last long so I had to think of something else to keep my mind occupied and keep the imps at bay. This was especially relevant at night, as the imps were most active when I was trying to sleep and kept me awake and uneasy. I was advised by doctors and nurses to play music to drown out the voices, which I did and the louder the music, the better the effect. It was particularly ironic, that Meat Loaf's 'Bat out of Hell' sent hell's own demons back there.

The Celtic Holy Grail Quest

Chapter 8 Dr Frankenstein Episode

Despite all my efforts with music, research and exercise, my condition continued to deteriorate and eventually I was readmitted to hospital. My time there was very dreamlike as I was sedated most of the time. All food tasted of cardboard. Some of the medication dried my mouth out so much so that my tongue literally stuck to the roof of my mouth. I felt totally detached from reality. All the doctors, nurses, patients and visitors appeared as actors and actresses following a script. My demonic companions and I were the audience watching them play. I didn't interact with them, I just watched the actors and actresses take the stage and perform the hospital drama 'Down and out in Ward A44.' During this time I slept, listened to music on my Walkman and received visitors to my hospital bed, where I had become a recluse.

My appetite diminished, until I was eating hardly anything and I lost weight, becoming emaciated. In my partially starved state, unusual visions became predominant and I started to see all manner of demons and predators from the spirit world. For that was what I was, prey for malevolent spirits to stalk and drag back into their dark underworld, cold and dank with the smell of death. I would often glimpse a dark lake and hear the cries of the drowning souls as they sank beneath the oily black surface. I could feel them pulling me there and would be found screaming by

David Stocks

the nurses as the black wraiths tried to engulf me.

Despite my exhausted state, I was eventually tempted to go for a walk with some other patients and nurses. I had found exercise did my spirit good in the past and decided to give walking a go, in spite of my exhausted state. The weather had finally taken a turn for the better and we walked around the nearby university park. We circumnavigated a beautiful lake, where swans basked in the sun, which shone down on me and filled me with its positive energy. The walk, sunshine and exercise invigorated my being and I returned to the hospital in a better frame of mind.

With exercise came the return of my appetite and I soon began eating more, with ever more frequent bouts of exercise to keep my system energised.

It was shortly after this that I had my review with a consultant, who decided that I was now well enough to be released from hospital. Initially I felt better, but when the weather changed for the worse and I stopped going to the gym, the improvement became short lived. The imps once more began their taunts, especially at night:

'He cannot hide in the darkness, but others can.'
'Everybody hates him, there is no wonder.'
'There is no light in his soul, only darkness.'
'It is from darkness he hath come and it is to darkness he shall return.'

The Celtic Holy Grail Quest

I took to turning my light on, as night-time and darkness was one of my childhood fears resurfacing in my time of discontent. The light, however, only cast shadows around the room. I imagined malevolent creatures hiding within the dark recesses of these shadows, waiting for sleep to take hold before devouring me - if I was foolish enough to close my eyes - releasing my subconscious mind and opening the portal to night's demons. I entered a semi-conscious state, neither asleep nor awake. The whole world seemed blurred at the edges, where a shoe would metamorphosise into a creeping black claw and then back into a shoe again, while my ears would be continually assaulted by the demons' hideous whisperings.

It was in this exhausted, frightened and self loathing state of mind that I visited my psychiatrist. He recommended Electronic Shock Treatment (ECT), which passes pulses of electricity through the brain, to shake the brain and jar it into action. The theory is that it removes pessimistic thoughts, breaking down mental barriers and reconnecting positive pathways. But to me it sounded like a crude experiment, belonging to the 19th century and fiendish experiments performed on corpses, provided by the loathsome criminals that were the body snatchers.

ECT sounds great, doesn't it? Anyway, I didn't care; I was so depressed that I would try anything. The experience was quite surreal. I was led into an operating theatre and told to lie down on a bed. Beside the bed was a large metal machine, which was humming. A doctor approached me, who looked just like Dr Frankenstein, with a manic grin, white frizzy hair and a gleam in his eyes. He told me to relax while he attached the wires to me.

Relax? Yeh right! I'd relax while he attached what looked like jump leads to my temples, so that electricity could zap across my brain and rewire the inner sanctum of the temple of my mind. The leads had suction pads on and were attached with a special gel for better conductivity. When this was done, the white coated psychiatrist came and gave me an injection in the back of my hand. The last thing I remember before sleep took hold of me was his manic grin as he pressed the power button.

When I came round, I was groggy but felt alright. The first thing I did was go and look in the mirror. To my relief there were no scorch marks on my head. I didn't feel any different, but things seemed a little vague. I put this down to the anaesthetic. It was only as the days and weeks went by that I realised that large chunks of my memory had gone. There were entire holidays that I could not remember having been on amongst many other things. My memory was like an incomplete jigsaw with some of the pieces missing. As for my mood, it hadn't improved at all. So all that ECT had achieved, was to wipe large portions of my memory.

The Celtic Holy Grail Quest

I continued to be assaulted by voices, which along with Dr Frankenstein, I felt had been sent by some sort of demon. I imagined I was being watched all the time and often would see inky black shadows in my peripheral vision. These would be indistinct, fluid patches of darkness that would disappear when I tried to focus on them. I was becoming paranoid that it was all part of some demonic plot to destroy me and send me screaming down to hell. Wherever I went I was being watched, my every thought recorded. My every transgression was noted, I felt I was being led down a path to oblivion and sent signals that controlled me. My brain would periodically rush with electricity, like a static wave of energy. I came to the conclusion that I had been implanted with an electronic receiving device which was picking up these energy waves and processing them as instructions to control me, sent by the demon. Perhaps Dr Frankenstein had inserted this device during my ECT treatment? The whole world was against me; I didn't know what to do.

In every Grail romance there are villains that try to waylay you. Dr Frankenstein and his cohorts were knights of the order of the white lab-coat, the most devious and tricky beings ever sent to distract a true Grail Knight from his quest. I was not about to let them forestall me on my Grail errand and I carefully took up the trail where I had left off, peeling back the layers of Celtic mythology that contained the secret of the true Grail in their midst.

David Stocks

It was just a matter of determination and with mad scientists and hell's own demons at my back, I had plenty of that.

The Celtic Holy Grail Quest

Chapter 9 the Green Man

I was sent to see another psychiatrist, who reviewed all the notes from past consultations and analysed my symptoms afresh. She paid particular attention to the voices I heard and decided that these were the most incapacitating part of my illness. She diagnosed me with psychosis (where perception of reality is at fault) and prescribed me with new medication to tackle this. This slightly alternate perception of reality is of particular interest to me and forms one of the integral pieces that make up the jigsaw puzzle from which my Grail quest is constructed. Later in the quest the very nature of reality comes into question, at this stage all I can say is, 'What we perceive as reality is the greatest of all illusions.'

It was at this time that I started attending woodcarving classes at a place called SPAN (a centre for rehabilitating mentally ill people). The first project I tackled was the carving of the 'Green Man.' This rang a bell with me, for the image of the Green Man was one of the central figures in Celtic history. The Green Man is usually depicted as fresh sprouting vines and leaves, intricately woven into the form of a head, capturing the very essence of nature.

Carvings of the Green Man can be found in churches throughout Britain, dispersed amongst interlocking creepers and foliage, peering down

David Stocks

from roof bosses, screens and misericords; images with Celtic Mother Earth connotations, bearing little relevance to Christian beliefs. I had myself seen an impressive collection of Green Man carvings in a Chapter House in Southwell Minster, not too far from where I live. Southwell had once been part of Sherwood Forest, of Robin Hood fame, and it may be that his legend had its origins in the Green Man.

I undertook the carving of the Green Man with relish. As I chipped away at the wood, I imagined the Celts doing the same thing two millennia ago and the techniques they used then would not have been very different to those I was using at the time. Each strike of the chisel created one more detail of the carving; invigorating aromatic scents filled the air as the chisel bit into the grain of the wood. I could smell the scent of the Green Man that had been bottled up within the tree for centuries, waiting to be released. It felt appropriate to be carving the spirit of nature out of nature's own wood. From nature, nature's essence is wrought.

Carving is a thing of patience, as you cannot rush a carving. One inaccurate strike of the chisel and the carving is ruined. You cannot replace a piece once it is cut from the whole. From carving you learn patience. The sculpting of the Green Man reflects nature, for nature herself is patient taking many years to grow a tree. Why you ask, am I carving wood from a tree that has been felled?

The Celtic Holy Grail Quest

From my understanding of the Celtic way, the Celts believed in living in harmony with Mother Nature, making sure what they took from her was sustainable. I therefore took care to use wood from a sustainable source. Wood that had been cut to allow more space for other trees to mature or wood cut only where replacements had been planted.

And so, like a buried acorn that eventually grows into a mighty oak, a seed had been planted in my mind that would eventually germinate into a greater understanding of the Celtic way of life and their synchronicity with nature.

I had been taught a lesson too, one of patience, and I realised that the Celtic Holy Grail could only be found though patience and perseverance. The Grail was not going to give up its identity easily to me! If I was to find the Grail I must journey deeper into Celtic beliefs and carefully uncover any signs that I found on the way. Only by following these signs and fully understanding their meaning, was I ever going to achieve my Grail Quest.

David Stocks

Chapter 10 Gamelstune - Wheel of time

Another seed that was growing in my mind was the memory of that tortuous journey back from work and the unease conjured within me on arrival back at Gamston's moonlit village green in the dead of night.

Following a hunch, I embarked on research into the origins of Gamston. I visited the local library at West Bridgford and it was there that I found a leaflet that had been produced by Gamston and District WI. I discovered that Gamston probably originated from the Old Danish word Gamal meaning 'the old.' It was originally called Gamelstune and was listed in the Doomsday Book.

The words 'the old' sent a shiver through me, for in the presence of moonlight an ancient and sinister feeling pervades the green. What secret lay hidden in Gamston's name? The village centre held within its tiny boundaries, a source of great lunar power. What lay within this small triangle of grass that made up the village green? Gamston had its roots stretching deep down into history's veiled depths, hiding secrets as yet unknown.

Further investigation into moon worship and any associated cults was required, for it was obviously having a detrimental effect on me. Conversely the sun was filling me with its positive radiance when

The Celtic Holy Grail Quest

it shone. My health was inextricably linked to celestial bodies and the celestial forces they administered. This made perfect sense, for surely their presence has impact on the earth and all life upon it? Our ancient ancestors understood this but we, with all our science, are bound by scientific restrictions and will not speculate into a region not understood by modern science. Science is the new religion, populated by the scientific priesthood who are unable to see outside the narrow confines of their specialization and egos. As with most religions, they are unwilling to accept something that cannot yet be explained, refuse belief outside its own doctrines.

I took a more broadminded approach and undertook an intensive search through books on Celtic law and religious practices. I found nothing specifically relating to sun or moon worship, but I did come across ceremonies and festivals associated with the solstices and seasons.

To understand this we need to look at the Celtic view of time. The traditional Christian way of looking at time is linear. The book of Genesis starts at the beginning of time, while the revelation to John concludes with the end of time. Celts didn't concern themselves with the rise and fall of the Universe. They held a cyclic view of time, such as happens in nature: autumn-winter-spring-summer-autumn.

David Stocks

I was reminded of the shift in time I experienced as the black cyclist pedalled past me. Everything I did was in some way interrelated.

Was the black cyclist literally cycling through time? Riding some kind of diabolic steed, along the straight path of a ley line, wheeling back the hands of time? What would happen if he cycled in the other direction? Would time get caught up in the cycle's spokes and spin forward into the future?

The Celts celebrated festivals that corresponded with the beginning of each season:

- **Samhain** (summer's end) marked the onset of winter's months. October 31st is modern day Halloween. A time of great power when the real world and the spirit worlds cross.
- **Imbolc** (in the belly or ewe's milk). The time when the pregnant livestock would begin lactating, signifying the onset of spring, February 2nd.
- **Beltaine** (bright fire), May 1st., celebrated the return of the sun and the onset of the hottest time of the year.
- **Lughnasa** (Festival of Lugh), August 1st., marked the beginning of the autumn harvest period.

In between these festivals the Celts celebrated the winter and summer solstice and the spring and autumn equinox. A diagram of the Celtic wheel of time is shown below:

The Celtic Holy Grail Quest

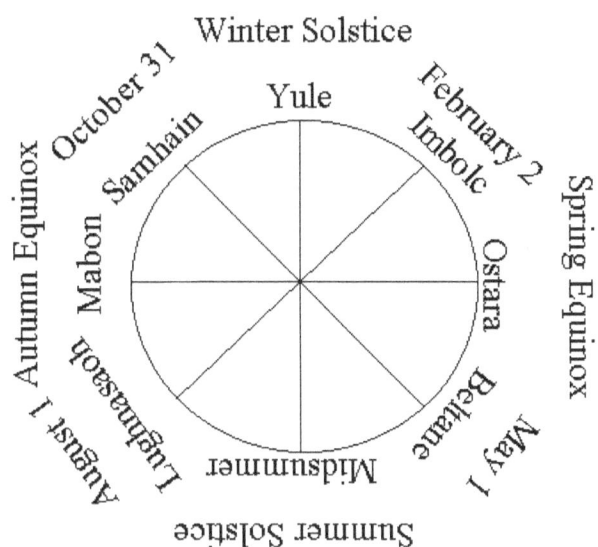

As you can see it really is a wheel of time and resembles a modern bicycle wheel or an older chariot wheel. The modern notion of time, with its circular clock face, owes no small debt to the Celtic wheel of time.

Could I take the cyclist's route and roll back time to before depression and psychosis descended on

David Stocks

me? Or roll forward time to the future? But what future had I got? Or even, how long had I got? One thing was for certain I could feel the passage of time in Gamston, or should I say, Gamelstune.

So as the clock ticked on I journeyed back in time in search of the Grail, to its ancient origins in the mystical land of the Celts. To attain the Grail, I needed to travel in the mists of time to a land in harmony with its people. I knew that the Grail was not going to be found in the present, corrupted and polluted by materialistic modern man.

The Celtic Holy Grail Quest

Chapter 11 Stoned Henge, Druids and all that

The voices and visions experienced solely by me and quite possibly the construct of my mind, the medical term for which is psychosis, I believe may have had a root cause in the so-called recreational drugs that I used during a period of time as a teenager. I did not experiment with these to a large degree and therefore cannot say that they have done me a great deal of damage, but I had one particular episode when I went to the Stonehenge Free Festival, that I was on a permanent high from the hallucinogenic effects of certain types of marijuana. I believe during this time I had some of the stronger hashish varieties, which may have affected me in later life.

At the time of my trip to Stonehenge Free Festival, I had a good friend who went by the name of Bod. Now Bod had persuaded me to acquire an old Suzuki 250 motorbike, of disputable background and of even more disputable road worthiness (it was a heap of junk!) The plan was to convert this wreck into a vehicle capable of transporting us to the said Stonehenge Free Festival.

Off to the breaker's yard and bike shops we went, with a list of automotive parts that Bod assured me would transform my dilapidated Suzuki into a roaring monstrous mean machine, the like of which had not been seen since the proverbial 'Bat out of Hell.' In preparation I grew my hair, donned

David Stocks

a worn leather jacket and wore oil stained jeans. That was it; I looked the part, one mean, grease-streaked biker. If anyone bumped into me in the street, they just knew I had the beast's mother-of-all motorbikes sitting in my backyard, or in this case a beat-up old Suzuki 250 that wouldn't start!

I was reminded of when I first got a motorbike, a 50cc Puch Monza. It was a nice looking bike, but being 50cc would only get to 40 mph and was small to boot. I took my first mean machine on a run from Nottingham to Hull to show my Granddad, a former rider of a Norton, a classic British 'cafe racer' bike. The journey took an age and having virtually seized up in the riding position, I stopped on the way in a little place called Market Rasen. This is one of those magical experiences in life, where time slips away and you are transported back to a bygone era, for having parked my bike I wandered round the corner to find a cafe with a horde of bikes parked outside. The cafe was heaving with leather clad bikers and their sexy chicks and there was a half moon jukebox playing in the corner. The style of everything: the cafe, the bikes and the people, harked back to the milk bars of the 50s where all the bikers used to meet. I whiled away an hour in there, taking in the scene and talking bikes. I told them that my phantom machine was parked around the corner, embarrassed to let on what it actually was. I completed my run to Hull and back, but have never since returned to Market Rasen. I have often reflected on that mysterious cafe in the

The Celtic Holy Grail Quest

many years gone by and I remain convinced that for that one brief period, I pierced a bubble in history and joined the milk bar bikers back in the 50s. For an instant in time I was Marlon Brando in 'The Wild Ones.'

At some point in everyone's lives, people see themselves as movie stars. Writing this account of my life and quest now is like unravelling fallen spools of film, threading them back on a projector and playing out the celluloid movie of my life on a silver screen, in which I take on various film star personas.

Returning to the main thread of this chapter, that of the heap of scrap metal roughly arranged in the form of a bike, Bod confidently assured me that we would soon have the bike on the road. Unfortunately he didn't have the mechanical skills to back up his impressive confidence. After a number of weeks, the appliance of all things mechanical, a few deliberately induced petro-chemical explosions (the only time the bike ever moved), we resigned ourselves to the fact that our trusty steed was not going to take us to Stonehenge, or even the end of the street for that matter!

I was impressed with Bod's friend's mechanical expertise however; he stripped down a motorbike and rebuilt it in the upstairs bathroom of his bed-sit. A motorbike was born in a blackened bath, a primordial soup of sprockets, gaskets, cylinder

David Stocks

heads, spark plugs and Satan's own engine oil. On the day of reckoning, he bump started it by riding it straight down a steep flight of stairs and out through the front door of his flat. The bike roared down the road and both bike and rider were never to be seen again. Now that's what I call a grand exit! Incidentally, the very same engineering genius was the friend who sold me my motorbike; it could be said that if he couldn't make it go, then we were never in with a hope.

Having no transport, next to no money, we were left with only one means of getting to Stonehenge in time for the Free Festival, that of hitchhiking. With much use of our thumbs we managed to hitchhike our way from Nottingham in cars, vans and lorries, eventually arriving on Salisbury plain and the site of Stonehenge Free Festival in a clapped out old Ford Escort. It wasn't the sixties, but at the time of Stonehenge Free Festival, it was once again a time of free love, peace and literally anything goes. As we drove into the hippy encampment, a thriving city of multicoloured tents, we descended into an herbal haze which stayed with us all weekend. Kids leaped onto the bonnet of the car and leaned in through our open windows, offering us all kinds of substances, most of which I had never heard of, from herbal additives to tobacco that I would soon be sampling. The weekend had begun.

At this time, one of the last years that the Free Festival ran (it was banned soon after), the police

The Celtic Holy Grail Quest

stayed well clear and the only form of policing was by the Hell's Angels. We pitched our tent - an amazing feat of structural engineering including combinations of poles, fabric, string, tape, wire, plastic, cardboard and carpet - never seen before or since. We settled down in our Shaman's hut and the weekend passed in a hallucinogenic haze. Trips outside were few and far between and although I only have vague recollections of that festival, what I remember most is the emphatic love and happiness that everyone shared.

A notable highlight of the weekend was when I flew higher than everyone else – literally! It was at a time when dangerous sports of the parachute kind were in their infancy and someone had a novel idea of towing a parachute across one of the fields from the back of a Landover. Having no fear of heights, particularly in my euphoric state, I volunteered for the ultimate trip. It was very windy the day I stepped forward for my journey into the blue yonder and all experimental flights were temporarily halted until the wind dropped. With the day drawing to a close, it was eventually decided that the wind had slowed enough (not at all) to make an ascent. I was first on the list and was soon strapped into a harness (probably before I came to my senses and changed my mind). With the hastily uttered instructions, 'Start running before you land,' I was dragged off my feet behind a rapidly accelerating land rover.

I soared in the air like an angel, underneath my

David Stocks

fiery orange canopy in the evening sun. I was flying over a psychedelic field of tents, drifting on heaven's own strings. My mind and body took flight. It was the ultimate trip, blowing on an herbal breeze over a sea of love. The fiery eye of the sun burned on the horizon as the land rover slowed down and I made my descent. Remembering my instructions I broke into a blazing run, my feet skipping off clouds of hemp smoke as I descended from the heavens, like the Greek god Mercury (messenger of the gods). Mother Earth came up to greet me and my flight from the heavens was broken as I tumbled head over heels across the field, ending up ingloriously tangled up in a heap of parachute silk and cords. I had been to heaven's own realm and returned with an important message to mankind: 'Don't go hitching rides behind out-of-control land rovers attached to a parachute on windy days, while high on a combination of substances of unknown origin!'

It was still an experience I wouldn't have missed for the world, but I was lucky to come out of it unscathed; it was perhaps because my body was in such a relaxed state that I didn't incur any serious injury.

Psychedelic rock legends Hawkwind played through the night and with dawn came the summer solstice at Stonehenge, an ancient monument whose stones had been placed in a precise way to observe the heavens and in particular, events such as the summer solstice. I

The Celtic Holy Grail Quest

could not get near the monument through the hordes of New Age revellers, but the moment was special, in the presence of the stones and the stoned. It was a feeling of universal harmony and love; I am not a hippy and have long since given up use of herbal substances, but it was the most genuine experience of my life and one I will never forget.

Being at an ancient site, long revered by the Celtic people and the Druids, on the most important date in the Celtic calendar, had a profound effect on me. It was an experience that was to be ultimately rekindled with my interest in the Celts in later life. Druids performed sacred ceremonies at the stones to welcome the sun back on that longest of days, their beliefs dating back thousands of years.

Here is a little bit of history on the Druids:-
Ancient Druids were first known to exist way back in history, approximately 4000 BCE. (The fascinating early origins of Druidism I will discuss in more detail later on in the book). Alongside Druids were Bards and Ovates. Ovates were the herbalists and doctors, valued members of Celtic society who were revered healers.

Bards were inviolate and could choose when and where they performed. As carriers of messages, news and important cultural information, the Bard's role was essential to the Celtic people. Bringing harm to a Bard was out of the question, for all contact with the outside world and tribal history would be lost.

An important role of the Bard was to maintain the connection with the otherworld, through a twilight state (dreamtime), where the boundaries between the corporeal world and the otherworld blurred. The best way to reach this twilight state is not through the use of hallucinogenic or psychotropic drugs, but to explore the hypnogogic state between waking and sleeping. I am writing this passage now, in this very state, barely awake, with dawn just on the horizon. Much of this book has been written in this state, usually in the middle of the night, in the semi-sleep mode of consciousness. In this altered state of mind, the otherworld is tangible; you can almost feel it, touch it. The Celts very much believed in the dualistic conception of the world, being that of the corporeal world and the otherworld. The otherworld is rarely seen, but rather felt as a sensation in the heart or body. The Bards duty was to convey this spiritual feeling of the otherworld in verse and music. The bard takes on the role of master storyteller and musician, a messenger from the otherworld.

The Ollamh is the highest degree of the Bard in the ancient Gaelic society and it is that of the Druid. The Druid performs highly spiritual forms of poetry and ritual, and tries to reveal the 'Poetic Truth,' the inspiration from otherworld Gods and Goddesses behind the poetry. The origin of the word Druid is thought to have been derived from

The Celtic Holy Grail Quest

DRU, which means Oak tree (sacred to the Celts). The Gaelic word Druidh has also played a part in the definition of the Druid, Druidh means 'a wise man' or 'magician.' This last interpretation fits in appropriately with the modern view of Merlin, thought to be a Druid and a Bard.

Druids believed in a supreme creative force, that of the Earth Mother Goddess and the Sky Father God. Druids' authority in many cases outstripped the Monarchs and they cast the final decision in many disputes. They were the sole interpreters of religion and had the power to excommunicate; the most horrible punishment of all, besides death.

I will speak more of the Druids' great power, beliefs and history later in the book.

I returned to Stonehenge with my then wife, Sue, on many occasions and pondered on these great stone monoliths, transported all the way from Wales for construction on this particular site. There must be a reason for this vast undertaking; through millennia we have lost the secrets that they conceal, lost the knowledge of how to use this powerful spiritual place. You can feel a sense of peace and oneness with this giant stone shroud, a connection with the infinite, through which universal mysteries lie.

My favourite standing stones, however, lie about eighteen miles from Stonehenge, at Avebury. These stand more naturally on top of circular earthen mounds, with rings of these mounds and stones lying within one another. There is such a feeling of peace at these stones and Sue and I spent many a sunny day wandering in and out of them, unhindered by throngs of tourists or security fences. One of the most remarkable sites at Avebury is Silbury hill, a prehistoric conical shaped mound 130ft high, the largest in Europe. It was never used as a burial mound and its purpose to this day is a mystery. Nothing is known of what may be contained within the mound; if anything, to me it is sacred and beautiful in its symmetry.

Menhir (standing stones) lie scattered across Britain and Europe and through extensive travelling with Sue I have been lucky enough to see many of these. Tombs of giants, massive beehive shaped chambers, prehistoric caves, all of them staggering in their scale and construction. A legacy of the past, a message for the future, but has mankind now lost the knowledge that accompanied these stones? In this age of science we seek in science to explain everything, we have lost that inner instinct that links us to the spirit world, where all the answers lie. We may have evolved to use tools and apply scientific methods to the problems of humanity, but in animals there still exists a greater understanding, one in which a higher spiritual connection is maintained, one that we have now lost.

In my quest for the Grail, I seek to re-establish that link, to reach a higher understanding and attain

The Celtic Holy Grail Quest

the Grail. One thing I know about the Grail is that it won't be found by looking for it directly, it can only be found through trial and hardship, by following the Celtic way.

Chapter 12 Major Oak

I was still being besieged by whispering malicious voices. My little demonic friends had taken to distorting my thoughts and working their own evil ideas around them. I would be thinking while wood carving and they would snigger in the background, saying malicious things to each other like, 'He's going to carve up his wrists, let's watch!'

Such sentiments obviously didn't raise my spirits. I decided I needed to keep myself occupied and get more sunshine, to try and keep the voices at bay. I volunteered for BTCV (the British Trust for Conservation Volunteers), who maintain the natural habitat around Britain.

At dawn I boarded a minibus full of volunteers and we set out to do some pruning and cutting back of trees to allow full future growth. We began in a small copse of trees in the Mansfield district of Nottinghamshire. Donning helmets and gloves for safety, we gathered an array of tools and ventured into the surrounding woodland. The task in hand was thinning: cutting down non-native trees from the woods to allow more light and space for the indigenous trees to grow. We divided ourselves up into teams of two and I was paired with an experienced conservationalist nicknamed, by strange coincidence, Bod! I was destined to know the odd Bod. He was about 22 years old, tall and thin with tanned skin and blonde dreadlocks; a

The Celtic Holy Grail Quest

nicer guy you could not possibly hope to meet.

It was early spring and frost sparkled on the branches like diamonds, picked out by the sun's dazzling rays as it sliced through the trees, forming crystalline patterns in the angular formations of the branches.

Our first job was to fell the foreign trees, which involved chopping out a V shaped groove low down on the trunk with a billhook (a blade, hook-shaped at the end, with a handle). The tree could then be felled with a hacksaw, using the notch as a starting point. When the tree was about to fall it was important to make sure that no-one was in the direction of the falling tree. To make doubly sure, we shouted 'Timber' in proper lumberjack tradition.

Bod pointed out the different types of tree to me, so that I could identify the native from the non-native trees, showing me bark and leaf shoots related to each different species. He went off to make tea, building a small fire in a clearing on which to boil the kettle. I went deeper into the woods in search of trees in need of clearing. Despite Bod's clear instructions I soon became unsure about which trees I could chop and which trees needed to be left. As I pondered the dilemma I found myself venturing further and further into the wood, although I didn't realise it at the time. I eventually decided on a tree that I thought could be cut down and set to work on it. As I chopped into the fresh green tree, sap oozed out of the cut, appearing like blood as it dripped over the copper coloured bark. A feeling of unease descended on me, but I didn't want to be judged a failure and so carried on with my hatchet job. It was only as I shouted 'Timber!' I noticed that everywhere had gone silent. No birds were chirping and I couldn't hear anybody's voice. Everything was deathly still.

Smoke had drifted up from the fire Bod had made and all I could see around me were skeletal silhouettes of the trees, dark and hazy in their gaseous shroud. Coughing I descended the slope in what I thought was the direction of the camp. The slope steepened and I tripped and fell over a tree root as my momentum took me downwards fast. Desperately I reached out and snatched at a branch, trying to stop my fall deep down to who knows where? The end of the branch ripped into my right palm and then sprung back, out of reach. Reeling from the pain in my hand I tumbled uncontrollably deep into a gully, cracking my head on a tree as I reached the bottom.

I came round after an indefinite amount of time and stumbled in a daze along the floor of the gully. The banks and trees swirled around me in my semi-conscious state. In the distance I thought I could hear a horn, resonating deep and low through fissures in the earth. I stopped still and listened hard. It came again, only louder, crashing like a wave upon me, the sound rushing through my bones, shaking them and leaving a cold

The Celtic Holy Grail Quest

unpleasant chill deep within me. What was this madness that had descended on me? A ghostly phantasm of the mind, brought on by concussion? The chill tightened its hold and fear drove my legs, staggering into a half run of their own compulsion. Again I heard the horn, the sound ricocheting off the gully walls, crashing onto my sides and making my run even more drunken.

I kept running, following the twists and turns of the gully. Again and again the horn sounded, ever more deafening, ever nearer. Who was this pursuer, from whom was I fleeing? Was he real or ethereal, a demon or a creation of my mind? Time had become warped and could no longer be measured. It was just an instant, yet an eternity since I had first heard the horn. How could I measure time when I had run so far and yet felt just a second pass by? In my current state, normal rules did not apply. It was like a lava flow with time split into a slower crust on top and quicker molten lava below. Time was moving in two streams and I was mixed up in both of them.

I hazarded a glance backwards and glimpsed a sight that sent an icy chill through to the marrow of my bones. Riding a chariot of living wood was a warrior with antlers growing from his head, his lips pursed, blowing a huge horn. Pulling the chariot were giant coal black dogs, their eyes glowing red, the very hounds of hell. The rational part of me attributed my pursuers as visions brought on by concussion, but it was my irrational side that took over. I was being hunted; adrenalin kicked in,

David Stocks

making me sprint with renewed urgency. I could now hear the howls of the dogs, mixing with the sound of the horn, resulting in a soul rending diabolic cacophony. I ran on and all the while the walls of the gully appeared to be contracting; lined with a dark green moss they pulsed in time to my ever faster beating heart. I felt I was running through some kind of giant earthen artery, being led to the heart of the forest, to a fate at which I could only guess. My legs were burning, my lungs on fire, but still my pursuers chased me deep into this earthen fissure. Focusing on the path ahead, I resisted the urge to look back at my supernatural pursuers and pushed on with every last reserve of my body strength. Just as my vision was starting to blur and I could feel myself on the verge of passing out, I staggered into a large clearing.

I stopped dead in my tracks. Everything became deathly still, in fact the silence was deafening after the wall of noise I had just experienced. In the centre of the clearing stood a tree that I knew well, the Major Oak, a tree that had stood for centuries, if not millennia. Deep down I understood that what I did next was vital, both for my life and my soul. Climbing over the fence that had been built around it, I approached the ancient tree, with reverence. The oak stood with stilts supporting its larger branches, like a bent old man on crutches, aged but venerable. My next actions were of utmost importance, not just for my life - for I could sense my hunters just beyond the edge of the clearing - but also for the life of the forest. Blood dripped

The Celtic Holy Grail Quest

down from my gashed hand and it was then that I knew what to do. Scanning the tree, I found a split in the wood, where a crack had opened. I stretched out my bleeding hand and placed it deep within the gap. Time stood still. I felt part of my life-force flowing out of me and mixing with the sap of the giant oak tree. I could feel my energy running down through the tree, deep into the earth and out through the roots of the tree. I felt foliage extending out from my body, my face, my hands and my arms; soaking up the sun, photosynthesising and energising, the sweet nectar of sap rising up through my veins, mixing with my blood, coursing through me. I was at one with nature and nature was at one with me. I understood at once the meaning of the Green Man; it was symbolic of the union of Man with nature, a Shamanic experience, an inner transformation that I was now undergoing. Through the roots and the leaves of the tree I was engulfed by the presence of the once mighty Sherwood forest, the legendary hideout of Robin Hood, who himself has been linked to the Green Man. This was a place of power, where legends were born and myths created. A place that must continue to be nurtured and venerated. A site of symbolic significance, where nature's heartbeat can be truly felt.

In a state of bliss, I drifted away from this world and slipped into peaceful unconsciousness.

David Stocks

Chapter 13 Time slipped by in the night sky

Darkness engulfed me,
Immersed and drowned me,
My mind taking flight,
Into the night.
Neurons fired,
My brain rewired,
Cosmic awakening,
Universe awaiting.
Solar winds,
Giving me wings,
Sending me sailing,
Through stars cascading,
In a galactic swell,
Where black holes dwell,
Spiralling downwards,
Chronologically inwards.
Time is space,
The universal case,
Interconnected,
Cosmologically accepted,
Slip through to infinity
And a parallel affinity.

The Celtic Holy Grail Quest

Chapter 14 Happiness Interlude

I awoke with a start, staring up at the leafy trees above me, lying back on my bed of moss. Everything seemed so vibrant and alive. My eyes had been shut, unable to gaze at nature's true beauty. Now they were open, as were all my senses. I could feel the soft sponginess of the moss, breathe in the fresh air alive with the scents of wood and leaves. I could hear the song of birds and the wind through the trees. Like a rush of adrenalin, nature infused me. This was more than just an awakening, it was rejuvenation, an earthly reincarnation, a flight of the soul, a body made whole.

Gone were my pursuers, the felling of the tree, adjudicated and forgiven with the advent of my union with the major oak.

Old man of the forest,
With his oaken heart,
Bowed with age,
Gnarled and bent.

A forest guardian,
Sherwood's monument stands,
Still dignified,
The lord of the dell.

I feel nature's essence,
Course through his veins,

David Stocks

And find understanding,
Deep in my heart.

In this kingdom of trees,
Sounds a solemn song,
So many have fallen,
From his mighty domain.

Whispering leaves,
Herald my companion's return,
From my woodland dream
I forlornly stir.

I couldn't explain my absence, for what could I say? I just said I had become lost and thanked them for finding me. It was only after an arduous trek back that I realised how many miles I must have wandered, with no sign of the gully that I had earlier traversed on the way back.

I went home with hope in my heart and no sound was heard from my demonic companions. Something inside me had changed and I did not want to lose this regeneration of spirit. With this in mind I set off for a bookshop, hoping to find a Celtic volume that could lead me on this new found path. While browsing the bookshelves in search of Celtic lore, my eyes alighted on a book called 'The Art of Happiness,' by the Dalai Lama. My Celtic quest was interrupted, for here was a text to which I could relate. This was a book with a simple philosophy: Look at the positive side of

The Celtic Holy Grail Quest

things and just be happy. Love everyone, even your enemies.

Using this philosophy I was able to maintain my high spirits. After a few weeks I was still in this mood when I received a call from another psychiatrist, who was keen for me to take part in a study being done on people who suffer from depression. I explained that I now felt myself free from its dark clutches, but he said that it would be useful for me to take part anyway and that he would like to see me to discuss it further. He was very friendly, about five feet eight inches tall, with dark curly hair and a thin weasel-like face and a Cheshire cat grin. I had to fill in a questionnaire and then he asked some further questions. He then told me that he thought that I was far from recovered as I had disrupted sleep patterns and racing thoughts, all indicative of severe depression. I agreed but it didn't stop me feeling good inside. He explained that he wanted me to do some audio-visual tests while wired up to an electroencephalograph (hundreds of pairs of electrodes attached to the scalp that record brainwave patterns). He then got me to sign a consent form for the test and a date was set.

On the day of the test I was greeted by Ilana, a Greek psychology student who was performing the tests as part of a research project for her PHD. Ilana was very pleasant and chatty. She was dark haired, olive skinned and had large brown oval eyes. She sat me down and showed me the equipment. There was a computer monitor on which my brain wave patterns would be recorded and another monitor with a seat in front of it, where I would be performing my interactive tests. Finally there was a computer from which hundreds of cables and leads extruded. I was initially sat in front of this array of wires which were all bunched up and interwoven, like a knitting pattern gone wrong. I was then introduced to the last piece of the jigsaw, something that I could only describe as a swimming cap with sockets. It was one that I imagine a hedgehog would wear, with all its bristles protruding from the multitude of sockets adorning the surface. For hedgehogs of the swimming persuasion, this was the ideal hat. With a smile and some gentle persuasion, I was coaxed into donning the cap and allowing the electrodes to be inserted. Prior to the insertion of each electrode, a gel was injected into the socket, giving better conductivity with the scalp. The sensation of the gel injection was quite extraordinary. It felt like the liquid was passing straight through the scalp and down through the brain, sending shivers into my cerebral cortex. Once the gel was applied, a numbered electrode was inserted into that socket and the process repeated on the next socket. Once I was fully connected I had wires shooting off my scalp in all directions, rather like Albert Einstein's hair. The whole process took roughly an hour, at the end of which I once again felt like part of some old Frankenstein movie. This time, however, they were only going to monitor, not fry, my brain.

The Celtic Holy Grail Quest

I was guided over to the chair in front of the monitor; trailing wires behind me, now interwoven in what I thought closely resembled the Celtic knot pattern. It seemed wherever I went, I would always be influenced by Celtic lore and motifs. Throughout the tangled skein of this story a Celtic thread wove its way, guiding me onwards to an unknown destination.

Once I was comfortable in the chair I was given a control pad with a series of buttons. I then carried out a set of calibration tests pressing the buttons, while Ilana recorded my brainwaves. Once Ilana was happy, we went on to the full tests. These included pressing a button corresponding to a colour flashed up on a screen. These were designed to test your reaction and accuracy. The same test was then repeated with coloured words written out in different colours e.g. **Yellow**. I had to press the key corresponding to the colour the word was written in and not the actual colour spelt by the word. In the previous example it would be the red key. From many years of working with computers, I had built up an empathy with them and I found I could pick up the colour that was going to appear, even before it appeared on the screen. It was like I was receiving feedback from the computer, through the electrodes attached to my scalp.
I did these and a number of similar tests and got a virtually one hundred percent success rate, in lightning quick time. This far surpassed any other

David Stocks

person's score. It was like I was floating in cyberspace where numbers, colours and words would flash up in my mind like neon signs. I became disconnected from my body and could feel the complex web of the internet all around me, all woven together in a never-ending stream of data, analogous to the never-ending pattern of the Celtic knot. The insight came to me again that everything was interconnected through some grand design, one thing linked to another and another, into infinity. The Celts knew this but modern man with all his science was only now beginning to understand it.

I left Ilana somewhat perplexed, but happy with how I had achieved such results.

Soon after these tests, I went with my wife to see a dance production at the local Nottingham Playhouse. One of the dances was set in a forest, with a hypnotic green swaying backdrop. In a trance-like state I had visions of white angels flying down from the balconies around the theatre.

> Surreal,
> Incorporeal,
> Angelic Host,
> Holy Ghost,
> Mental Protectorate,
> Psychiatric Directorate,
> Heavenly Vanity,
> Preserving my Sanity.

The Celtic Holy Grail Quest

I interpreted their presence as a call for me to help protect and save our forests.

My mood continued to be bright for a couple of weeks after this, but then it dipped and not just a little, for it dropped into a deep chasm, dark and lonely.

Chapter 15 Sinking in quicksand

Lonely was not quite correct however, for my demonic friends had returned with a vengeance. Their tirade of abuse resumed, with such delights as:

'He hath black blood, for the devil is inside him.'
'He doth not know how pathetic he is.'
'He hath but a dark hole for a soul.'

Back down the path of misery my assailants led me. The more I fought them, the more they preyed on me. Like quicksand, the more I struggled, the more I sank.

I was prescribed new drugs, which helped deaden the voices to a certain extent, but not totally. My mood did not lift until I started going for walks. The exercise, fresh air and nature revived my spirits enough to apply my mind to seeking work.

With the rejuvenating effect of the outdoors, I sought a job that would keep me close to that environment. Scanning the employment columns I eventually found a vacancy that matched my requirements. The post was for a Park Ranger, based at West Park, Long Eaton. I applied for the post and was pleasantly surprised to get an interview. I was equally successful at the interview and it was not long before I was starting a job as a Park Ranger. It was a seasonal job that ran from

The Celtic Holy Grail Quest

late Spring through to Autumn.

On the whole the job had the desired effect upon me; I got a lot of fresh air and sunshine and felt more energised. I was plagued at night by bad dreams though, demons trying to drag me down into hell's inferno. These dreams carried themselves over into the daytime and I was constantly on my guard, fearing I was being watched by some malevolent presence.

One of my duties included setting out the bowling greens and taking money for play on the greens. This at first didn't bother me, but my paranoia kicked in when I was on my own covering a bowls match. Everyone appeared in white coats that made me think of an army of psychiatrists and they were all making demands. I felt that they were out to get me and that they were in league with the psychiatrist who had given me the electric shock treatment (ECT). The whole experience proved too much and plagued by the cantankerous army of white coated bowlers, I was signed off work for a couple of weeks.

During those two weeks, my mind became detached from reality for large periods of time. Sleep brought troubled dreams that transformed into visions on waking. The boundaries between sleep and rousing blurred. I took to using my laptop computer to try and keep my mind focused, but this only made matters worse, bringing the digital world into my mental world. Now I was

David Stocks

haunted by binary ghosts, streams of 1s and 0s would flash on the screen and through my mind. I was now sailing in an electronic universe, a fusion of the neurons of my mind and the electrons of a computer. I could see the cosmos made up of electronic bits, everything could be broken down into individual binary units, switching on, off, on off 1, 0, 1, 0, 1010101010 …

… 10101010101 and every switch of 1 or 0 cascaded through the universe. Everything was connected; a change in one particle could be felt in every other particle, the universe. Therefore the universe could be understood by looking at one particle, the universal building block.

My head swam trying to contain the ideas that were flooding into it. While emptying my laptop case one day I came across the screen dump that I had made that night I had left work and entered my altered state of mind; the night that my Celtic Holy Grail quest began. I could now see binary digits as something that needed deciphering. With this in mind I set about decoding the screen dump, to see if any patterns or meaning could be gained from it. I was seeking order out of chaos, little did I know what I was going to find!

I looked at it and realised that on closer examination it was not totally random and that the same groups of binary digits kept recurring. These were:-

00100, 00101, 10110, 01001, 01100 and

The Celtic Holy Grail Quest

01000, 00101, 01100, 01100.

I had the sense that there was a message there. But what was it? Or was I imagining it?

I took each binary number in the first group in turn and translated it to its decimal equivalent. To do this you place the binary digits under the corresponding decimal row of numbers, starting at 1 and doubling up to 2 then 4 then 8 and 16 onwards. So the first row of binary digits would line up like this:-

16	8	4	2	1
0	0	1	0	0

To get the decimal number add up all the numbers with the binary digit 1 underneath. In this case it is just 4, so the decimal equivalent of 00100 is the number 4. On this basis I worked out the rest of the numbers in the group, as shown below:

16	8	4	2	1	Decimal number
0	0	1	0	0	4
0	0	1	0	1	5
1	0	1	1	0	22
0	1	0	0	1	9
0	1	1	0	0	12

I now needed to translate the numerical data into alphabetical. To do this I substituted the decimal number with the corresponding letter of the alphabet. The position of each letter in the

David Stocks

alphabet is shown below:-

A	B	C	D	E	F	G	H	I	J	K	L	M
1	2	3	4	5	6	7	8	9	10	11	12	13

N	O	P	Q	R	S	T	U	V	W	X	Y	Z
14	15	16	17	18	19	20	21	22	23	24	25	26

A chill went through me as I spelt out the message hiding underneath the binary code, for out of chaos comes the lord of darkness, hidden in a string of numbers, malevolent and watching me:-

16	8	4	2	1	Decimal number	Letter
0	0	1	0	0	4	D
0	0	1	0	1	5	E
1	0	1	1	0	22	V
0	1	0	0	1	9	I
0	1	1	0	0	12	L

Dare I decode the next string of numbers?

The demonic voices whispered their insidious messages in my ears.

'The lord of darkness doth await your soul.'
'He hath no pity for such a low and worthless soul as yours.'
'He awaits your fearful fate.'

Haunted and taunted I set about decoding the

The Celtic Holy Grail Quest

second string of numbers, with some trepidation.

16	8	4	2	1	Decimal number	Letter
0	1	0	0	0	8	H
0	0	1	0	1	5	E
0	1	1	0	0	12	L
0	1	1	0	0	12	L

The message was clear, the devil was coming to take me to hell! The demons on my shoulders reaffirmed this.

'Hell awaits, no soul can escape its grasp, especially such a lowly one as yours.'

'The chasm opens, death calls, step over the edge into the eternal fall through hell.'

It appeared that the bottomless pit awaited me. It was calling me and I could not escape its malignant grasp. I should kill myself now and get it over with, but I couldn't. Something was stopping me. Somewhere deep down inside was a spark of hope, that if rekindled, could light and lead me out of my despondency.

More through despair than hope I re-analysed the last code, this time decoding the digits top to bottom, and I was somewhat staggered by the result:

David Stocks

	16	8	4	2	1	Decimal number	Letter
8	0	1	0	0	0	8	H
4	0	0	1	0	1	5	E
2	0	1	1	0	0	12	L
1	0	1	1	0	0	12	L
Decimal number	0	11	7	0	1		
Letter	0	K	G	0	D		

There as clear as daylight I could see the letters G-O-D: GOD. I did not know the significance of the letter 'K' before the word 'GOD' or the relevance of zero as the letter 'O', but the word just jumped out at me and further investigations would reveal the meaning of the whole code.

What however did God have to do with hell? Surely God's realm is heaven and hell is the most ungodly domain of all? I then remembered that everything that had happened to me so far was of Celtic origin and so it was to the Celtic myths and legends that I once again looked.

Next I made a startling discovery; delving into the

The Celtic Holy Grail Quest

history of the Celts I found that they were originally referred to by the Romans and Greeks as the Keltoi. This became the name for the people from then on. This name has changed over the centuries until it was shortened to Kelt right up to the 20th Century, with books in the 1920s - 1930s referring to them as 'The Kelts.' It now became obvious that the 'K' in front of GOD in fact referred to Ketoi or, in modern terms, Celtic God. But what of HELL?

Hell is also known as the 'underworld' or 'Abyss.' In Celtic legend, 'Annwn' or 'the Abyss' (the underworld) is not a place of eternal suffering but rather quite the opposite; it is a land of joys and marvels containing a magic cauldron of rebirth, the land of the Celtic gods. This cauldron gave rise to later legends of the Grail. So this code was making a direct referral to my Holy Grail quest, a quest to be reborn in spirit and soul, to wash away the contamination of my old life and start afresh! Maybe I should be looking into the Celtic underworld, or 'otherworld' as it is also known? I was on the trail; little did I know where it would lead me.

David Stocks

Chapter 16 Nurture Nature

I returned to work with renewed hope, but no longer took on any duties on the bowling green. I now had a focus for my Celtic Holy Grail research into the depths of the underworld, in search of the cauldron of rebirth.

My work around the park took me a lot closer to nature. All around the park were trees. One part was like a mini arboretum, a winding path of trees, each one different, wending their way through the park. While I was in the trees I could hear whispers, but these were not malicious whispers, but rather the sweet rustle of wind through the leaves; a sonic tonic. In the trees my stresses would disappear and my mind relax, entering mental freefall.

>Drifting leaves,
>On a gentle breeze,
>Branches swaying,
>Can you hear what they're saying?
>This is nature's language,
>Of the Environmental Age.
>Industrial pollution,
>Brings environmental revolution.
>Listen to their song,
>It won't take long.
>This world is choking,
>While your engines keep smoking,
>Slash and burn,
>Make earth an urn.

The Celtic Holy Grail Quest

Fire is not the answer,
It gives the planet cancer.
Ozone depletion,
Solar radiation,
You will all fry,
Through this hole in the sky,
Don't burn oil or coal,
And widen the hole.
Nurture nature,
Don't rape her!

Initial bliss turned to anger: Why are we destroying this world? Is nature's beauty lost to everyone? Are we blind to the fact that the planet is going to die or are we just closing our eyes and pretending that it won't happen? I could now understand the source of my mental afflictions. My body was in tune with an ailing planet and I could sense the cancerous plague that was attacking it. Greed had overcome humanity and humanity was using earth's resources without any thought for the consequences. I understood that this had to be stopped and that the cauldron of rebirth was not just a quest for *my* rebirth, but the rebirth and healing of the planet. I was a modern day Knight in search of the Holy Grail and the Holy Grail was closely linked to the regeneration of the planet! But I also knew there was a great force of evil trying to stop me.

The Holy Grail takes on many guises: It is a chalice containing Christ's blood, a cauldron of rebirth, an endless supply of food, a provider of

David Stocks

wisdom. It is not any one thing and cannot be obtained by those directly seeking it, in any of its forms. To know the Grail is to get one step nearer to achieving it, but such is the nature of the Grail that every step you take towards it is one step further away.

The Celtic Holy Grail Quest

Chapter 17 The Abyss

It's peculiar the path we tread, for when the underworld is mentioned the abyss comes beckoning. I fear what I don't know and the world surrounding death gives no clues to what lies therein. It is a world that can only be conjured up in the imagination, a fantastical world of heavenly bodies or fearful demons, depending on your slant on life. So no sooner are the halls of death decrypted, than I am brought closer to that realm through my work as a Park Ranger. One of the duties that entered into my work repertoire was the unlocking and locking of the cemetery gates, close to West Park. When arriving in the morning I had to unlock the gates and when leaving at sundown I had to lock the gates.

On unlocking the gates one morning, a mist enveloped the ground and spread out around the gravestones, so that only the tops of them were showing. The gates swung open with a groan, the sound dampened by the mist. I looked round at the cemetery and saw a woman dressed in funereal black; with the mist covering her feet she appeared to hover between the gravestones. With a shudder I turned around and headed on to West Park.

It wasn't until later in the day that I remembered the incident. I returned to the cemetery just as the sun was setting. It balanced on the horizon as a

David Stocks

fiery red ball and there silhouetted against it was the same woman in black. This time the haze from the sun obscured her feet and I watched her glide across the graveyard to the chapel at one side of it, entering within. I followed her in, for I needed to tell her that I was locking the cemetery and she would have to leave.

Stepping into the chapel, which was only small, I looked around for the mourner. She was nowhere to be seen and despite a vigilant search, I could find her nowhere. There was no place she could go, no crypt, no other exits. I was mystified and I felt a chill go right through me, even though it was a hot summer's day. I opened the door to go back out of the chapel and a black cat scuttled out from behind a pew. Was it just chasing a mouse or was it a creature of darkness and what, if any, relationship did it bear to the woman in black? Shivering I went back out and locked the cemetery gates. A black cat can bring luck, it can also be a portent of death!

Death was quick in coming; I had no longer slipped from consciousness than I was caught in a crossfire, taking a bullet full in the chest. Bizarrely I felt no pain just bemusement as to what was going on. I floated above my body and could see my lifeblood pumping out from my heart. My assailants were just chatting as if nothing had gone on. I could feel myself being dragged down a tunnel of darkness, white light shining around the edge. Surrounding me I could hear the voices of

The Celtic Holy Grail Quest

my demons laughing, enjoying my discomfort as I descended into a bottomless black hole, a void for my soul. The ever consuming void engulfed me and I lost consciousness again.

Rays of warm light embraced me. Up above the sun shone, its healing energy infusing and spreading throughout my body until I could feel it shining from within, burning bright and strong. Every part of my person was filled with energy and I felt a great joy inside. Something inside clicked and I understood the power of the sun and why the ancients worshipped it. I was in solar rapture, a state of bliss …
… I awoke drenched in sweat and burning up from the heat of my dream. I could remember it clearly and knew that I was being given an important message, one which I could almost grasp. Something about light from darkness, but what could it mean? I had been led to believe that if you die in a dream, then this is your deathbed and you never wake up. I now knew this not to be true and to die in a dream was to experience something beyond that which can be seen in the waking world.

I had descended down to the lowest depth and only at this lowest point had I been given the highest understanding and the gift of joy. How I wanted to reconnect with this joyous feeling!
I had experienced the healing power of the sun; the Grail is said to have great healing properties. In one of the Grail romances the Fisher King is

David Stocks

healed by the Grail and his land that had been made barren is made whole again. Could the essence of the sun be captured within the Grail?

At this stage of my quest, I was encountering more questions than answers.

The Celtic Holy Grail Quest

Chapter 18 Charnel House Phantasmagoria

After a brief return to work, I felt that a change of scene would do me good and I decided that a visit to Austria would be just what I needed. My parents have an apartment above the lovely old mountain town of Schladming, high in the Dachstein-Tauern region of Austria and it was to there that my wife and I retreated.

Stresses and strains disappeared with the invigorating mountain air and scenery. All thoughts of a Celtic Grail quest were temporarily suspended, as I enjoyed summer walks across mountain meadows and cool trails through pine scented forests, where deer would spring from behind trees and birds of prey would hover overhead.

We sipped beer and Gluhwein in cosy mountain huts, whose timbers were old and gnarled, of ancient origin. Living in this region of Austria was like going back in time, unspoilt by industry and technology; in much of the area the way of life was the same as it was hundreds of years ago. Garlic and herbs hung from ceilings and hay stooks (hay drying on poles in the ground) that stood like little people or lines of scarecrows on the mountainside.

We made many excursions from Schladming, one of our favourite being to Gausausee, which is a

David Stocks

lake high up in the mountains on the other side of the Dachstein - the highest mountain after which the region is named – a place of great beauty, particularly early in the morning.

We set off for Gausausee at dawn one day and arrived there at about 8 am. The lake had a surreal quality to it. A layer of mist floated over the water, sparkling in the early rays of sunlight. It appeared as a scene from an Arthurian legend, in which a hand holding Excalibur rose up from the depths of the lake. I was reminded of the Grail quest or rather my Celtic interpretation of it. The mist imperceptibly cleared to leave a stunning site, the lake became a giant mirror and lofty peaks all around it were reflected deep down in the lake's surface. The image was crystal clear, not a ripple disturbed the surface; with the blue sky above and the encircling crown of mountains this was surely heaven's mirror and we were just pilgrims at some holy place. The sunshine was a welcome break from previous days of heavy rain deluging the area and there was a freshness in the air as the sun heated the damp earth. Invigorated, we decided to venture on to the smaller upper lake, Heuter Gausausee. The trek to this lake was on a winding path through thickly scented pine trees. The earth was a damp and springy mossy carpet beneath our feet. Birds sang their morning songs in the branches above. The whole place had an enchanted feeling and we felt privileged to be treading the soft path through this emerald green forest of tranquillity. The path twisted and turned

The Celtic Holy Grail Quest

sharply as we ascended higher. It was on this steep stretch that we met an old lady who was bent over picking something from near the base of a tree. She was hunched, with a heavily arched back, her face wizened and bearing a crooked nose. Her apparel was a long patchwork skirt, her shoulders covered by a shawl. In one hand was a basket into which she placing the proceeds of her picking. Her manner, her dress and whole look gave the appearance of a witch, yet on our approach she looked up and gave a friendly smile holding out her basket to us.

Beckoning for us to approach, we stepped up and examined the contents of the basket. Within it there was a collection of tiny yellow mushrooms, the like of which I had never seen before. Saying nothing she offered us some mushrooms from her basket. Warily we took a few and thanked her. Having done so she beamed and walked off down the path. I wasn't sure what to make of the whole encounter, but the feeling of the place was pleasant and I was sure that there could be nothing nasty within such an environment. So perhaps rashly, I took one of the mushrooms and placed it in my mouth, onto my tongue. It tasted of earth and loam, small but succulent, arousing curious sensations within my palette. Without realising I bit into it and my mouth was flooded with juices that were surely greater than the capacity of the mushroom. My taste buds were awash with a most peculiar combination of flavours, both bitter and sweet at the same time,

David Stocks

quite unlike anything that I had sampled before. I chewed and my mouth tingled inside with this newfound flavour. Swallowing I felt the tingling sensation spreading throughout my body, until my whole being became alive with electrical pulses radiating out through my nerve fibres. My brain too was swamped with this sensation. Neurons cascaded around my grey matter firing jets of energy throughout both hemispheres and out through my skull. This energy connected me externally to my surroundings and I could live, feel, smell, taste and hear everything around me in a much more complete way. I was one with everything and everything was one with me. Strange musings came upon me:

> Am I thinking these thoughts,
> Or are these thoughts thinking me?
> Never did the real,
> Seem so surreal.
> I feel so small,
> Yet never so tall,
> A microscopic spec,
> On an interplanetary trek.
> A cerebral journey,
> A quest for learning,
> A cognitive void,
> My mind overjoyed.
> Playing the fool,
> A learning tool,
> Cosmic speculation,
> Mind inhalation,
> All is one,

The Celtic Holy Grail Quest

And one is none.

What did these thoughts mean and where were they coming from? Everywhere around me I could see interconnections. The whole world, the entire universe was a puzzle, where every piece interlocked with every other piece. If one tiny particle changed then every other particle in the universe would also be changed.

Interconnectivity is the glue that holds everything together. I believe that one way or another everything is connected to everything else. Taking Newton's law of force one step further from:
'For every action there is an equal and opposite reaction.'
To a more general event driven formula:
'For every event another event is triggered.'

With these thoughts in mind we arrived at our destination. The trees cleared to leave a bowl scooped out of the mountain range, into which a lake had been poured. The lake had flooded with the recent rains and covered the surrounding meadows with an inch of water. The effect was mesmerising; the verdant green grass glistened under water and a multitude of colourful flowers sparkled like precious jewels, as the sun shone through the water. The flowers reminded me of stars, twinkling in the night sky, the vastness of the universe captured within this small lake. It was a mere glimpse of what lay beyond, a tenuous link between nature and the heavens, yet I could see

David Stocks

the heavens mapped out before me in my mind's eye.

We sat like gods on a rock above the lake, transfixed to the spot for an indefinable time and it was with great reluctance that we finally left this special place. Our descent back down was in a semi wakeful trance and we arrived back at our car before we realised it. We then made tracks for Hallstaat, a place with strong Celtic roots, for it was here where many of the earliest Celtic archaeological finds were unearthed.

Hallstatt tumbles down a mountainside into a lake, which reflects its image deep into the waters below. The houses perch precariously on the steep slopes of the mountain, the staggered roofs appearing like steps down, spires jutting out tall and proud; a picture postcard image of a town steeped in history.

We wandered into the town, through narrow alleyways, over bridges and across churchyards, until we came upon a charnel house. This was a resting place for bones, exhumed from the churchyard after 10 years to free up space in that hallowed ground. Entering the charnel house was like stepping through a gateway, passing into the transitory world of the deceased, this side of death's realm. Inside illuminated by dim candlelight, were hundreds of skulls with bones stacked beneath. What made this scene of phantasmagoria even more impressive was the

The Celtic Holy Grail Quest

paintings on the skulls. Each skull is painted with the name of the deceased, dates and flowers or foliage of some kind. There were two skulls sat next to a cross with snakes painted on them, weaving in and out of the eye sockets. These are representative of the serpent in the Garden of Eden and of original sin.

> Silent skulls survey,
> Their sacred domain,
> Where wanderers stray,
> To view their remains.
>
> Icy fingers reach,
> In this skeletal hold,
> In search of a soul,
> In death's darkened hole.
>
> Garlands and wreaths,
> Adorn the dead,
> Ivy and oak leaves,
> Interred from their beds.
>
> Do not dwell,
> In this spiritual home,
> Or the dead might take you,
> For one of their own.

The experience of visiting the charnel house was deeply moving while chilling at the same time. I sensed the souls of the deceased at peace but there was also a chill and a tug on my soul,

David Stocks

beckoning me across into a transitory world between the living and the dead, one short step from death's own gate. The empty eye sockets hypnotised me, the snakes on the skulls near the cross slithered in and out of the eye sockets and their jaws. The candles cast shadows on the walls, thrown from the morbid tourists visiting the charnel house. These flickered and distorted on the curved interior of the crypt, wavering in the darkness like inky black demons reaching out to clutch my being. These phantasms and the staring skulls led to panic within and I beat a hasty exit.

Next we ventured up to the Dachstein ice caves, set high up in the mountains above Hallstatt.

Entering the caves was like entering a giant cathedral of ice, formations of which arched high up into the caves' recesses, bold pillars of ice transparently supporting the jagged ceiling. Sunlight streamed in through the entrance and the light danced about the cave refracting the spectrum of colours hidden within the beam and displaying them in a swirling kaleidoscope within ice pillars of light.

> Sunlight falls on God's frozen prism,
> Scattering into fragments of colour,
> A kaleidoscope of frosted light,
> Captured within a cathedral of ice.
>
> Sculpted glacial angels fall,

The Celtic Holy Grail Quest

Vibrating with the frequency of light,
Casting heavenly tears into crystal pools,
Mirrors upon celestial planes.

Anointed in radiant light,
Bathed in a tumbling rainbow of hues,
Spilling out onto golden shores,
Kissed by liquid sunshine.

In the birthplace of the Celtic people, I experienced a transformation of being. Enveloped in an array of light, I journeyed back to the Celtic home. Returning to this heartland, I was now equipped for the journey ahead and trials of mind, body and spirit that awaited me on my Grail quest.

David Stocks

Chapter 19 Badlands

The Autumnal days were starting to draw in on my return from Austria and the light cast was darker, with everything taking on a dull grey hue. I returned to my job as a Park Ranger, but my spirit was broken. I could not see any brightness in the future and what's more, I was assigned the worst of jobs, that of the dog run! This involved emptying the dog bins around the borough of their smelly contents and loading the said contents into the back of a pickup truck. Not only was this job undesirable in the hygienic sense, but it was also a very difficult job to navigate on your own. Finding hundreds of dog bins in the labyrinthine tracks, alleyways and footpaths of the Erewash borough was not an easy job. It was a task that filled me with dread. Each day I had to cover a different part of the borough and each day brought a different challenge.

Whatever they paid me was never going to be enough as I started my first day of the dog run. Following maps with all the strategic locations of the dog bins marked on them, I set off in pursuit of my malodorous targets. When I say strategic, I mean strategic in the fact that they were hidden away in remote places, down footpaths, in bushes, behind toilets, along snickleways, in fact anywhere difficult to find and access via a pickup truck. I wended my tortuous way round the first day's route with difficulty, finding the bins and hefting out

The Celtic Holy Grail Quest

their rancid contents into the back of the pickup. Progress was slow and the stench from the back of the truck grew as the day wore on. A good sense of smell was not a key attribute to have when doing this job. There is nothing more fetid and putrid than a truck full of dog dirt. My view of dogs turned from lovable creatures to annoying shit dispensers, whose sole purpose in life was to make mine more miserable. With a full load I came to my last pickup of the day. It was a bin situated by a canal, underneath a bridge. The only way to access this was to drive the truck off the road, over a curb, down a steep grassy incline and along a narrow canal footpath. With my heart in my mouth I swung the steering wheel round, mounted the curb and then pitched down the treacherous incline below. The truck wobbled and threatened to tip up as I skidded down the slope, my breaks doing very little to hold the momentum of my descent down. It was as I was trying to regain control that a giant black hound leapt out in front of me, making me jar the steering wheel and send me careering towards the canal. Applying all my force to an opposite lock and jamming on the brakes I screeched to a halt underneath the bridge, losing half of my noisome load in the canal, leaving one wheel hanging over the edge. Gingerly I put the van back into gear and inched it back onto the path. Deeply shaken by the experience, I returned to the park with the remnants of my load, the image of the giant black dog etched deeply into my brain.

David Stocks

Each day brought more unpleasant experiences, one particular incident being that while emptying the bin near a playground I was taunted by kids chanting 'Smelly, smelly dog shit man.' This knocked my self-esteem; how much lower could I sink than emptying bins of dog dirt? Not much! To make matters worse the voices in my head took up the chant, 'Smelly, stinky, pooey, no-good dog shit man'. It was demeaning enough doing it, without others rubbing it in as well.

This latest experience took me down to new depths of depression and it was in this state that I did the final day's round of dog bins in an area called Cotmanhay, in the suburbs of Ilkeston. As I drove into Cotmanhay, the buildings gradually became more and more dilapidated, until I turned off from the main road and entered a desolate area of boarded up derelict buildings, hundreds upon hundreds of them. It was a modern suburban ghost town. Everywhere was spookily quiet, not a soul entered this area, not a living soul anyway. Boards flapped in windows, Coca Cola cans rattled down empty streets, like urban tumbleweed. A feeling of oppression descended on me as I snaked my way in and out of narrow alleyways and I could feel thousands of eyes watching me. I had entered a domain disconnected from reality, from which the hard square-cut breezeblock buildings exuded a deep malevolence, a harsh coldness that had caused the original inhabitants to flee.

The Celtic Holy Grail Quest

I soon lost my way in this grey concrete otherworld and I followed the twisting and turnings of the streets with growing panic inside me. It was with some surprise as I exited one such street, that I found myself driving down a slope into a giant wasteland. Stretched before me was a mile wide stretch of hollow forsaken badlands strewn with twisted metal, tearing up through the earth and clawing at the sky from Hell's domain below. A putrid stench permeated the air, overpowering even the smell in the back of my pickup. Broken glass lay scattered everywhere, like shattered tears of angels. Lonely in one corner of the wasteland stood a rusty pram, its inhabitant long since exported to safer climes. I drove on into this barren area, fearful for my vehicle, but more so for my soul. This was the land of the desperate, which reflected my mood with chilling clarity. It was as if I was meant to be there. My self loathing and dark depression suited this bleak landscape; here was a rightful home for my soul. A scratch of colour caught my attention, the only colour in this desert. It was the red of a solitary dog bin, to which I was drawn with chilling inevitability. On approaching the bin the rancid stink became all consuming. All other senses reeled by comparison; the only thing I was aware of was the overpowering fetid stench emanating from the bin. I knew deep down that this was one dog bin I was not going to be able to empty, for this was the bin for hell's own hound. The excrement contained within smelt of fear, decay and lost hope. I spun the wheel of the pickup and put my foot down on the accelerator.

David Stocks

Tyres spinning in the dirt I drove madly out of the Badlands and away from hell. In my rear view mirror I could see a giant black hound silhouetted on the horizon. It did not move, yet all around me I could hear the savage panting of a huge dog in pursuit; a pursuit that led me back into the maze of derelict buildings, a maze that I must escape. The voices in my head were whispering 'Flee, flee all you like, but it is impossible to escape me.' Undeterred I kept my foot down and wove my way through the streets, knocking over trash cans and careering off railings along the way. I tore through abandoned streets not knowing where I was going. Forlorn houses soon gave way to grassland. Still I could hear the panting and howls of the giant hound behind me. I kept my foot jammed remorselessly down on the accelerator. Ahead a canal came into view, but as fast as I drove the hound continued to gain on me, yet still no visible presence of it could be seen in my mirrors.

There was one way across the canal and that was via a steep hump back bridge. I slammed on my brakes just as I reached it and the whole truck tilted skywards as I ascended the slope. The truck lurched, leaving the ground as it crested the bridge. For one heart stopping moment, it felt as if the whole vehicle was going to tip over backwards, before the front end dropped down and it flew down the other side of the bridge. In a cloud of dust it came to a halt just before a hedge. With the crossing of the river the sound of pursuit

The Celtic Holy Grail Quest

disappeared. It was as if the devil hound could not cross the water. Somewhat dishevelled I followed the footpath along the canal to a main road and used my road atlas to find my way back to West Park.

Whether the hound was something conjured up from my tortured imagination, I shall never know. This was not the first time I had been hunted though and I was beginning to believe I was up against forces employed to keep me from my goal. This only hardened my resolve and made me more determined to complete my quest for the Grail.

David Stocks

Chapter 20 Hemlock stone

It was during a respite from the dog run on the other side of Ilkeston, that I encountered the Hemlock stone.

Having yet again become lost, I had driven out of the Erewash borough and into Broxtowe. With lunch time long since due, I stopped at Bramcote park. Taking my sandwiches with me I made my way along a footpath I felt myself drawn to, a sign above the path signalled my destination: The Hemlock stone.

I crossed a busy main road and walked upwards, over an embankment and into some woods. The atmosphere at once became peaceful. I was surrounded by oak trees and heard a multitude of birds singing their songs. All was tranquil and I felt a deep inner calm inside, far removed from the sound of traffic I had just left behind.

It was in this untroubled state of mind that I emerged out of the woods and was confronted by the towering form of a rock before me. What made it so impressive was the way it stood on a grassy slope all on its own, no sign of any other rock formations. To me it looked like a whirlwind spinning up from the earth, the narrow first third being of red rock and the second two thirds like two twisting black storm clouds, one capping the other. The striations of the rock were speaking of

The Celtic Holy Grail Quest

age, like the wrinkles on a venerable old man's hand.

It was a clear blue sky and I leant back against the rock bathed in a pool of sunlight to enjoy my sandwiches. I soon slipped off to sleep, my mind spiralling with the patterns of the stone.

In my sleep the rock was brought vividly to life; it loomed over me dark and brooding, menacing and threatening. A full moon cast a shadow, a dark image of a giant anvil adrift on a silvery plane. I could hear my heart beating against the stone, all else was deathly still. What awaited me here this moonlit night? I tried to get up, but could not move. All energy had been drained out of my legs and I sat there fearful of what was going to come next. For something was going to happen, I could feel it in the air. My skin tingled and I could taste ozone on my tongue. But still silence ...

... Time ticked by as the earth rotated around the sun and the moon rotated around the earth. I could see it all as a giant clockwork mechanism with all the planets, the moons and the stars interacting with each other, forming a giant universal machine on which mankind was like particles of oil on one of the smaller cogs. In this I got a brief glimpse of infinity, but it was way too much for my mind to cling on to. The universal clock wound on and with it came dawn ...

... The sun crept up over the horizon behind the

rock and the sky burned a deep fiery red. The stone cast its anvil shadow, but this time a furnace glowed all around it. Upon the anvil a molten rod was placed, which was forged into the shape of a man. A giant hammer thundered down and smote it into shape. Once the blacksmith god had performed his work, the man stood up and I found myself in his place stood on top of the hemlock stone. I felt fresh, revitalised and newborn. I stared out at the surrounding countryside with new clarity. Everything: The grass, the trees, the birds, were all bursting with life I had never noticed before. I could feel nature about me, on me, in me and through me; coursing through my veins, running through the earth, soaring through the sky.

In this blissful state I woke up, feeling rejuvenated and more intimate with my surroundings. The sun was still shining on me and a fresh breeze blew through my hair.

Again I felt the Celtic past calling to me, a message cast in stone in the rock that I lay back on. In a dream I had sampled the power and beauty present in nature. I realised that modern man knew nothing of this and through power and greed, sought to destroy the beauty that nature had built. Forces that should not be tampered with would ultimately be mankind's downfall, for Mother Nature was a generous creator and a wrathful taker. What is given can be taken away.

The Celtic Holy Grail Quest

This great rock, alone on a hillside, cast from the realm of gods, stood there, a signpost on my quest for the Grail. In reading this sign and interpreting it, I took another step on the path towards the Grail.

This experience aside, the dog run was not a feature of the Park Ranger job that I enjoyed and it was for this reason that I was not sad, when at the end of the season I was not kept on. I left West Park changed for my experiences as a Park Ranger and I had plenty to reflect on in the months ahead.

David Stocks

Chapter 21 Lost days, endless nights

From working long days I was suddenly left with time on my hands and no idea what to do with it. I half-heartedly trawled the local newspapers in search of jobs, but my heart was not in it and I gradually became more withdrawn, cutting myself off from society. I kept myself occupied by taking long walks and exercising at the gym, but all the time the voices plagued me, taunting and mocking me:-
'He doth seek employment, but who would have such a worthless soul?'
'Look at him, no friends, all alone, what a pitiful being he is.'
'The devil has marked him and is waiting.'

My mind was constantly on the go, always dwelling on things and pondering. At night I would awake alert, unable to sleep, thoughts racing through me. Sometimes they would be negative thoughts, sometimes inquisitive, more often a mixture of both. I took to writing my thoughts down, trying to gain a better understanding of them. These would take the form of plain text or as in the case below a poem:-

Midnight Ruminations

Alone in my midnight garden of thoughts,
The moon casts shadows on my soul,
In knowledge lies my salvation,
False whispers are my damnation.

The Celtic Holy Grail Quest

I cast myself adrift amongst the stars,
Sailing with a cosmic goal.
On stellar winds my mind does fly,
Asking the question, who am I?

Material forged from immaterial parts,
A substance of thoughts made whole.
Am I part of a galactic computer?
A universal binary commuter?

White noise surges like waves,
Tossing and turning in a universal bowl,
Complex patterns are caught in the hiss,
They interlace in a numerical kiss.

The double helix of DNA strands,
Like a Celtic knot, sketched in charcoal.
Systems of infinite complexity,
Yet of subtle underlying simplicity.

Understanding is gained through trials and torments,
Wisdom found within a black hole,
In the beginning, there was an idea,
But from where that came it is not clear?

And so the routine continued; exercise - be it walking, the gym or tennis - was my salvation from the voices during the day. I pushed myself to the limits to keep them away and was soon in peak physical condition. At night voices would intrude on my sleep, but it was my active mind that would keep me awake and it was during the night-time that I would analyse, philosophise and debate ideas and problems in my mind. The day was a time for tuning my body and the night for tuning my mind. I felt that I was honing myself for some challenge, sharpening my mind, body and spirit ready for the onset of darkness. I was preparing myself against the forces of evil that I believed to be within myself, purging myself of them - either that or die in the process.

> I dwell in a dark pool of sin,
> Into which my soul is cast in,
> Sinking slowly forever down,
> I feel my spirit steadily drown.

In a desperate effort to break out of this negative cycle, I focused again on my Grail quest. I revisited the Grail legend and its roots in Celtic mythology. There are several references to cauldrons in Celtic mythology that have various properties, those of providing limitless food (god Dagda), as a source of wisdom and inspiration (god Ceridwen) and with the magical ability to revive the dead. All these are known Grail properties.

Grail legends speak of a wounded king ruling over a ruinous wasteland. This could be the Celtic God Bran who was king of Britain and as legend tells it was wounded in a war with the Irish. He instructed his followers to chop off his head, which then continued to live for several years. When he

The Celtic Holy Grail Quest

eventually died his head was buried under Tower Hill in London, as a talisman to protect Britain from invasion. In such a wasteland Dormarth (Death's Door) the dog acted as gatekeeper to the afterworld. This could explain the black hound I had seen. Was I ready to cross the threshold to the afterworld, for only through death could I pass Dormath and reach the underworld beyond? It is also said that underworld hounds run down and punish the guilty. This is the realm of the Celtic goddess, Cailleach. A destroyer (or crone), she is also known as 'The Veiled One.' She signifies the death of all things, the winter, the waning of the moon, preceding regeneration through her cauldron of re-birth. Through death and regeneration, would I reach the land of Tir Taingire, or was there another path to follow to find this mythical otherworld? Death came to obsess my mind and in my sleep it would haunt me. One such dream is described in a poem below, in which I encounter the grim reaper and feel his touch, a touch so evil that I woke up screaming.

Feast of souls

A twilight supper,
An Autumnal feast,
An old man hunched over,
He could be deceased.
A black cloak his cover,
All wrinkled and creased,
A stale dusty odour,

David Stocks

The stink of a beast.
With a curl of his finger,
He reaches out east,
Making me shiver,
His touch I want least.
Lost in blind terror,
All movement has ceased,
For it is the Grim Reaper,
And my soul is his feast.

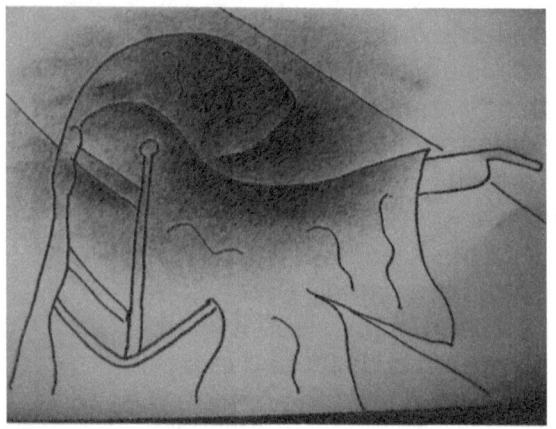

(Sketch I made of the Grim Reaper following the dream).

The next series of events took a peculiar turn. Whilst looking for references of dogs, I stumbled upon the word 'dogma' in the dictionary, one of the references being: a definite authoritative tenet. I wondered what the Celtic dogma was and scoured my books for Celtic dogmas. This in turn led me to find an entry for Ogma, the Celtic god of eloquence and literature; he is also the creator of

The Celtic Holy Grail Quest

the Ogham script. Ogma is known for his strength and fought many great battles. It is said he resides underground in a sidh called Airceltrai.

Ogham script can be used as a divination tool; it consists of characters made up from a pattern of lines. Each character represents a tree. These characters are found on ancient stones throughout the British Isles. The characters carved on sticks can be used as a divination tool by mixing them up in a bag and concentrating on a problem, then drawing one out. The rune corresponds to a tree and the associations and meanings suggested by the tree. I tried this method of divination and drew out the 'R - Ruis/Elder.'

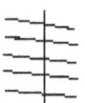

'Flow with universal energies to manifest healing and transformation.'

I meditated on the meaning of this rune and let my mind wander free from my bodily constraints, in search of the correct translation of the oracular advice.

Pushing outwards, I left my body and drifted on winds, the nuclear energy radiating from the sun, sending me out far into space. Planets I passed, satellites of the sun, orbiting and revolving in the dance of the spheres. Sound doesn't travel in space, but the music is always there. The sun is just a chain reaction, life on earth but a product of this. Mimicking the sun is the earth's inner fire, its molten core, energy as yet untapped by man. Volcanoes spew forth this energy from within and yet, has man tapped this power? Not now, not ever! So deep down my thoughts drift, through caverns untold. I sink slowly within the earth's fold. Wherever 'The Grail' is, I sense that it lies underground and that is where Man's future is to be found.

Keeping this in mind, I turned my research to underground places, of caverns untold and the secrets that lie beyond. Sifting through the historical notes on the subject, I found reports of 19th Century adventurers, who had reportedly found entrances to this great underworld located right here in Britain, one up in Yorkshire and one down in London; however, the exact locations were not revealed. I also found that many other religions place their otherworlds underground. In fact this is such a common theme throughout the world's religions that I wonder if such a place actually exists, a common root of most religions?

My quest takes me downwards in search of an entrance to this otherworld and I can think of no place better to start looking than in Nottingham, which has an extensive cave system.

The Celtic Holy Grail Quest

In this green land, somewhere beneath my feet lies the world's greatest treasure. I feel humble and undeserving of such a great prize. What right have I to lay claim to the Grail, when so many noble and worthy people have failed in their quest for it prior to me? I knew that I must not seek it through greed or avarice, for to do so is to fail. I must shed myself of all the burdens of the self and the corruption of modern man. I must travel as the fool and the beggar. The way of the fool is not what it seems.

David Stocks

Chapter 22 Masquerade

Before continuing my research on the Celtic underworld, it reached that time in the calendar when I lost another year to age. Another year wiser? I wish - wisdom doesn't come with age - as the antics of my forthcoming party shows. This as it happened was my 40th Birthday and I was determined to give the big V sign to middle age, believing that you are as old as you feel, so I threw a big party at my friend Ade's house.

Ade and his wife, Ita, have been long time friends of my wife and me. Ade is a bit of a character; you could describe him as an ageing hippy but he is far more than that. He has an open-minded outlook on life, he is very intelligent but doesn't like to brag about it. He is a laid back, fun loving, music mad, party fiend, born again pagan, with a suspect interest in toilet humour. Ita is lovely, petite and charming; how she ever copes with Ade's antics I will never know.

Ade and Ita have a fabulous house, which just happens to have a barn in the garden, the venue of many a wild party. We decided on a theme for this party of a Venetian masked ball, of the Rock'n'Roll variety. All the guests were invited to come in masks, not to cover up their ugly faces (in most cases), but to act out the carnival held in Venice every February; parading through the mysterious waterways lined with frescoed palaces,

The Celtic Holy Grail Quest

towers and domes (Ade's barn), dancing to the finest music of the period (Punk, Grunge, Rock and Ska). What truer reflection of the grace and finery of Renaissance Italy could we portray?

Adorned in my Phantom of the Opera mask (a white mask that covered a cross section of my face that I believed accurately reflected the duality of my nature, with the covered side being the dark side where my demons dwell) and Sue wearing her cat mask (reflecting her love of the feline kind), we made our grand entrance to the ball. Entering the barn (little Venice), we found the lights dimmed and were transported back through the centuries, to find ourselves wandering the magical alleyways of Venice. One wall of the barn was adorned with glittering masks, from which illuminated eyes peered at us. On the other walls hung scenes of Venice, the Bridge of Sighs, the Rialto Bridge and St Mark's Square. We were truly transported back to the baroque architecture and renaissance buildings of ancient Venice. These backdrops had been made for us by Phil and Jill, friends of Ade's and ours. I particularly hit it off with Phil, as you will see later in this account.

A marvellous cake had been made by my brother-in-law's partner, adorned with theatrical masks. Without much further ado, I strode over to the back of the barn and plugged my mp3 player into a power amp and the party began to the discordant, dulcet, harmonic and wailing voice of Kurt Cobain (Nirvana). Venetian dreams and

David Stocks

Rock'n'Roll themes. A party from the basements of hell, to the pavements of St Mark's square; a party of fire and light.

Demonic masks cavorted with instrumental, golden and glistening compositions. Inhibitions were lost behind the false facade of the masks, and the revelry continued unabated. Drink was plentiful and there was music for every taste, with different themes playing throughout the night.

The night progressed with the revelry spreading outdoors and a huge bonfire being lit. We danced around the fire like some ancient Celtic festival, adorned in our masks. As the fire started to dwindle, Phil and myself took to running across the middle of it via a hastily thrown down plank. Plumes of flames and sparks soared into the air. Inside the song Firestarter issued from the power amp.

The party was still in full swing when I retired to bed, never being one to last the night out even at my own party. Now although this was my party, I can only say I played an innocent part in the following affairs, as I was asleep at the time. A good friend of Ade's, who shall remain nameless for the purpose of this book, had spent the evening (supposedly) chatting to another female friend with the net result that the husband of this woman became irate at the attention she was receiving. This resulted in much ranting and raving. The word 'witch' may have been

The Celtic Holy Grail Quest

mentioned at one point; of course I am only recounting this tale second hand, so I may not have my facts right. Counsels were had, in which the injured parties had their say, to which Ade - ever the diplomat - managed to insult all and sundry. Having woken again, probably as a result of the conflicts going on downstairs, I eventually managed to stir and return to the party. By this time all the goings on had finished, the relevant parties had returned home and I was related this story. Not letting it spoil a good party, we stayed up until dawn and partied the night away.

The fallout of the party I am not going to relate here, but it makes a very amusing story. The net result being, that poor Ade, ever the champion of a good party, has not been able to hold another party since. I will say that there have been many smaller gatherings that have resulted in memorable nights at his abode.

Masks and costumes have played an important role in Celtic religion and traditions. One such tradition that I believe has its roots in Celtic festivals, is one that I witnessed by chance in Schladming when on holiday during the Christmas New Year period. In this a man dressed as St Nicholas was accompanied by young unmarried men known as buttermandl or krampussen, who wore furs and ferocious masks. They cavorted through the streets of Schladming at night, stretching their hideously clawed hands out toward the crowds in the streets. It looked like one of the

David Stocks

scenes from Dante's inferno. Cowbells chimed, creating a cacophony of sound. They are said to bring good luck and punish the idle. I must have been idle at that time, as it was around then that my first depressive moods started and I have been punished ever since.

The Celtic Holy Grail Quest

Chapter 23

Much as masks conceal the identity of their wearers, the Celtic Holy Grail contains many secrets within its legend and as such, so does this book. Hidden within the chapters and text of this book are various secrets. These must be deciphered and interpreted by the reader in order to obtain the Grail and understand its nature. Many of the secrets are linked by coincidences, a central theme that runs throughout the book. This book may also be referred to as 'The Secret of Coincidences.' Read on carefully for all is not what it seems. A number of significance is referred to in this self titled chapter, that of 23. A great deal has been written on this number and films have been made on the subject. It is a number of great power and is shrouded in mystery. Dip your toe into the pool of coincidence, magic and intrigue associated with this number and watch where the ripples flow in the fabric of space and time. For those who have not sampled the effects of the number 23 let this be an introduction; for everyone else may I bring further insights. I intend to broaden the horizons of phenomenon associated with the number 23 and bring it into the context of this book.

I will start with the title of the book 'The Celtic Holy Grail Quest,' which has coincidently 23 characters (note the title was created prior to the concept of this chapter). The alternate title suggested in this chapter, 'The secret of coincidences,' also has 23 characters. As you can see, 23 had great significance to this book right from the outset.

My birth date in European format is 22/10/1965. If you take the digits of the day, 22, and month, 1, and add them together (i.e. 22+1) you get 23. Another coincidence is that Jules (who will be a later part of this quest) would inadvertently regularly glance at the clock at 22:10 or 10:22; this was before she knew my birth date.

During the course of my Celtic research, I recently acquired 'The Druid Animal Oracle' by Philip and Stephanie Carr-Gomm. Druids have strong Celtic links and the Animal Oracle represents 33 of the most important and sacred animals of the Celtic and Druidic tradition, in the form of cards. In this pack of cards I was drawn to one in particular, that of the raven. This was a bird of great significance to the Celts, its jet black colouring gave it associations with death, but it was also known as a prophetic creature. I mention the raven in this chapter, as the page number in the 'Druid Animal Oracle' on which it appears is 66. The association with 23 is not immediately obvious, but if you take the numbers 2 and 3, then divide 2 by 3 you get .66 recurring, taking away the decimal point leaves 66 or page 66.

Further elaborating on the significance of .66 recurring, 666 is the mark of the Devil; the raven is said to be one of the forms the Devil takes. The

The Celtic Holy Grail Quest

raven has strong connections with the Celtic underworld - it is said to be able to cross between the physical world and the underworld, journeying into its darkest depths to bring back messages from the underworld. It is within these dark depths that I hope to find the Grail.

Further Celtic connections can be found with the Welsh god, 'Bran the Blessed.' After a battle with the Irish, Bran's head was decapitated and became an Oracle. Eventually Bran asked for his head to be buried under White Mount, which is now Tower Hill, where it remains to this day. It is said that as long as his head remains buried facing Britain's foes, then Britain will not be defeated. Bran is a Celtic name for raven or crow. The ravens on Tower Hill remain today as a defence against invasion. A little known fact is that Winston Churchill became a Druid prior to becoming Prime Minister and that when the ravens on the Tower of London were scared away by bombings during the second world war, Churchill had the ravens replaced by ravens from the Celtic heartlands of Scotland and Wales. I have also coincidently just visited Tower Hill on a trip to London; again this was before I knew anything about its association with ravens.

Ravens are also blessed with an uncanny intelligence; in another coincidence I have just read an article in Scientific American magazine that examines the ability of ravens to apply logic to problems. Ravens are able to solve tasks in lightening quick speed that they have no previous experience of in the wild. They have also been proven to recognise features of other ravens and human beings and distinguish between different people and birds. This article appears on page 46, a multiple of 23. I bought this magazine on the way to London, where I was staying at a hotel situated by Tower Hill.

In Cornwall, King Arthur is said to live on in the form of a raven until the time he is reunited with his kingdom as its sovereign. It is said to be unlucky to shoot a raven. The connection with King Arthur also ties in nicely with the Holy Grail quest, with the medieval romances of the Knights of the Round Table and their quest for the Holy Grail. Interestingly Druids gather in circles when meeting or performing ceremonies. The circle is of great significance to Druids and may have played some part in the legend of the Knights of the Round Table.

As previously mentioned, the Celtic way of life is to live in harmony with nature. I have highlighted the destructive way of modern life, with the resulting carbon emissions depleting the ozone layer. A study carried out by the University of Central Lancashire in 1999 calculated that 23 trees would need to be planted each year to offset the average adult's carbon emissions. Even within the environment 23 has significance.

The Celtic Holy Grail Quest

Of relevance to the Grail quest and mentioned in a number of accounts of the number 23, is the Order of The Knights Templar. This Order served under a total of 23 Grand Masters until its dissolution by Philip IV of France and Pope Clement V. The Order was originally founded at the Temple of Solomon and was called 'Poor Fellow-Soldiers of Christ and of the Temple of Solomon.' It became popularly known as the Knights Templar or the Order of the Temple. Its original headquarters was at the temple of Solomon, during which time they were rumoured to have unearthed a great treasure that some say was the Holy Grail.

One final look at the number 23 brings us to the concluding chapter of Genesis, chapter 23. This is deeply associated with death and the burial of Sarah. I will say nothing more on this topic now, but further reading and decoding of this book expands on this subject with profound consequences.

David Stocks

Chapter 24 The Celtic Knot and the Double Helix

You can't examine Celtic lore without inspecting the Celtic knot. The intertwining of the knot in its infinite loop to me looks remarkably similar to the interconnecting strands of DNA, which form an elegant double helix. Did the Celts two millennia ago know something about the fundamental building block of life that we with all our science have only just discovered? I wonder if there is some code to be unlocked within the Celtic knot?

What could be the key to matching these structures and unlocking the code hidden within? For one thing the Celtic knots can be more than two strands and can become quite complex in the patterns tightly interwoven, while DNA can branch off to become new DNA strands. This doesn't stop them both being one structure, no matter how many branches and turns they take.

I discovered that if you transcribed these patterns onto the rim of a wheel an infinite loop would be formed. If the wheel was then spun round, a continuously flowing pattern emerged. All the twists and turns revolved in a pumping action, like a machine. One Celtic knot I drew even looked like heart with blood pumping to and from it. From within the Celtic knot beats a heart and from this, life. From the strands of DNA comes the structure of life. They both had links to life; although the

The Celtic Holy Grail Quest

Celtic one may seem tenuous it is a regenerating code that works like an eternal machine when spun on a wheel.

From this I derive the following conclusion: Life is a wheel that starts slowly when we're born and then builds up momentum as we reach adulthood, before slowing back down as we get to old age and finally stopping.

This fits in with the Celts' view of the cyclic nature of time. The wheel or circle once again plays a central role in understanding the Celtic way of life. The Celtic knot and the circle, having no beginning and no end, represents an eternal cycle. The seasons of the year come and go, again in an ever repeating cycle. Like a Celtic knot on the rim of a wheel, the Celtic labyrinth takes the traveller through the twists and turns of life, eventually finishing life's journey back where it started from.

Time is not linear, rather cyclic in nature. By starting from the hub of the wheel of time it is possible to take a journey to any point in time, by simply travelling along one of the spokes from the axis to the rim on which time flows.

David Stocks

Chapter 25 Reflections of a Fishmonger

The crisp cool days of winter ended and with the approach of spring I felt a lift in my spirits. Daffodils bloomed in golden abundance and as the seasons turned, so did my life. I felt invigorated with the spring sunshine and encouraged by its glory I sought work again, this time at the local supermarket. I applied for a job in the bakery as I have a love of bread, but was significantly surprised when I was offered a job as a fishmonger. This was not a role in which I had imagined myself, as fish was one of my least favourite foods and smelly to pot.

Despite the upturn in my health and fortune, I continued to suffer from psychotic episodes.

One such incident occurred early one morning. I was walking across the supermarket car park towards the rear entrance and was just approaching the entrance when I heard footsteps running up behind me. I assumed it was someone who wanted to get in when the door opened for me, but when the door opened and I turned round to see who was there, there was no-one to be seen. This made me feel deeply chilled.

I clocked on and went to work on the fish counter. The first job I had to do was shovel bucket loads of ice onto the counter. The night crew had music playing and as I started shovelling a Ska track

The Celtic Holy Grail Quest

started playing, 'One Step from Beyond.' This is excellent ice shovelling music and I scooped the ice out while thinking of the earlier incident and singing along to 'One step from beyond.'

It was while working as a fishmonger that I came across references to a tradition of Celtic poets/seers. (In Celtic society, poets and seers are the same thing, interchangeable). The tradition states that poets must seek the Salmon of Knowledge to gain inspiration. Irish poets are said to be filled with Imbas and use the unfolding metaphor of a salmon thrashing upstream to spawn. To posses the Salmon of Knowledge is to possess the wisdom and beliefs of the ancient Celtic world. To touch or eat the flesh of the Salmon of Knowledge is to gain knowledge of everything in the world. The Salmon of Knowledge is said to have been imbued with these qualities after eating the nine hazelnuts from the tree of wisdom hanging over a pool in the otherworld.

Figuring I could do with some inspiration and knowledge in my quest for the Holy Grail, I decided to take advantage of my role as a fishmonger and hunt for the Salmon of Knowledge. It seemed fate had taken a hand and guided me to this unexpected vocation, for the one thing a fishmonger does come into contact with is salmon, multitudes of them!

There would be around five or six boxes of salmon delivered every day, each containing approximately four large salmon. That's over twenty salmon a day and they all had to be filleted. As you might expect, we got sick of the sight of salmon, so it was with much surprise that my colleagues found me volunteering to do the salmon filleting and undertaking the job with enthusiasm. I did notice they didn't do much complaining about it!

So I took to filleting the salmon but unknown to the other fishmongers, I was actually looking for the Salmon of Wisdom. I wondered what would identify such a salmon. It must be pretty distinguished, I thought. I started holding them up to the light, to see if the scales would sparkle with a magical light. I stared into their blank white eyes to see if I could see wisdom reflected in them. I even quartered and dissected the heads of the most promising looking salmon, those that intuition told me could be the ones, or had a certain shimmer to their scales. I don't know what I expected to find in such fishy dissections, maybe nine acorns instead of a brain!

Of course my colleagues started to give me sideways looks; this was not normal fishmonger behaviour, neither was it normal behaviour! I tried to explain with what I considered was an experienced fishmonger air, that I was grading them for quality in order to sell the best fish at premium prices or to give them to our most valued customers.

The Celtic Holy Grail Quest

Ok, I can hear you saying, 'How do you explain the dissections?'

There was an answer for that one too! I knew of certain customers who asked for fish scraps to use as fish stock. Salmon heads made particularly good fish stock if chopped up.

So there, I had the answers, although I still got some odd looks. What really tipped the fishy scales of me being 'one salmon short of a fish-counter' was the latest habit I had acquired, that of sucking my thumb. Now I really must explain at this stage, before you put this book down and lose all faith in me, that I had very good reason for doing that.

In Irish mythology there was a famous seer called Finn whose name means 'the wise or knowing one.' It was said that he gained his special ability while cooking a salmon: he accidentally burned his thumb and stuck it in his mouth. Instantly he knew everything in the world, because the salmon was the Salmon of Knowledge. So there, not so stupid after all!

However, this didn't stop my colleagues and customers thinking that I was 'away with the fishes.'

At the end of each day, I would leave the store covered head to foot in salmon slime. People went

out of their way to keep upwind of me; there was a funny smell in Gamston and it was me.
I eventually had to give up my pursuit of the Salmon of Knowledge as I didn't like the reputation I was getting and didn't want to get known as the local fool. One piece of wisdom I did gain from all this was, 'A wise man doesn't stink of fish.' I now pursue the Salmon of Knowledge purely in the metaphorical sense, swimming up the stream of life in the search of inspiration.

Having given up my physical pursuit of the Salmon of Knowledge, I found time for contemplation in between serving customers. As my mind drifted, I went through a philosophical period and ideas came upon me in abundance.

I believe it is only through having experienced so-called-mental-illness that I have been able to gain these insights. Below are some of the musings that I have had; while they don't directly relate to the main story, they reveal the growth in my mind, spirit and the transformations that have been undertaken.

Art

Intelligence opens the door to a multitude of things, one being art.

One of the beauties of art is all the forms it takes. Art is everywhere, in nature for instance: in the beauty of flowers, the grandeur of mountains, the

The Celtic Holy Grail Quest

patterns in rock formations, the web of a spider, the feathers of a peacock. Art can be appreciated by all the senses, in the sound of a music composition, the flow of water, the feel of silk and suede, the texture of wood grain, the poetic verse, sculpture, painting, photography, the scent of a flower or newly mown grass.

What if I could create some form of art that reflected my experiences since I became depressed and the thoughts that surround those experiences? Below is an outline of one such concept.

I wanted it to interact with all the senses and to convey to people my experiences, both good and bad. My idea was to build a sculpture, consisting of a crystal skull; in this skull would be a circuit and a mini radar dish. In front of the skull would be a screen.

The audience would interact with the art via a control panel to the side of the skull; this panel would be made up of a number of buttons labelled as follows:

Voices: This would make two demonic heads pop up either side of the skull; they would then be heard whispering into the ears making various derogatory comments.

Visions: The eyes would project images onto the screen of various visions I had seen that could not be rationally explained. They would be projected from inside the skull in order to differentiate from real images seen from the outside in.

Dreams: Again, images would be projected from the eyes but also sound and music would be heard, recreating some of the dreams that I have experienced.

Signals: A hissing wave sound would be heard, the lights would flash on the circuit board inside, the mini radar would spin round and binary images of 1s and 0s would be projected onto the screen. This relates to surges of electricity that I receive sometimes, pulsing across the brain. It can feel as though I am receiving a signal from outside and that I am being programmed to do something.

Tranquillity: Visions of snow capped mountains in the background with a cascading waterfall in the foreground, tumbling into a pool in a little forest glade. The sound of rushing water would be heard and scent of fresh pine smelled. This is an idealized scene of tranquillity and is a place I try to take myself when I want to relax.

Touch: This is not a button but a curved piece of wood. You run your hand from one end of it to the other, starting off with a highly polished smooth surface, progressing onto an undulating surface, then to a surface covered in soft fur that vibrates as you pass your hand over it, and low purring can

The Celtic Holy Grail Quest

be heard.

Time Lapse: When I was working on the fish counter there were occasions where what seemed like a minute in time was, in fact, an hour. Where had that hour gone? I know I am not the only one to have experienced this phenomenon, so what is going on?

It could be that your conscious mind has been transported to another place during that hour and your body is operating on your subconscious mind as an automaton. Where your mind goes during this period, I don't know, but it could be like computer software downloading. Periodically your mind may need a programming update. These updates may be essential to your life, helping you to adapt to change. It is only recently that I have noticed a time lapse again. I thought at this time depression could be a failure in the brain to download the latest code and therefore be unable to cope with the changes that life brings.

I am adding this last paragraph as a footnote, some time after completing the chapter. While I was adding more content, I noticed a distortion in the current subheading. The words 'time' and 'lapse' appeared on two different levels, both on the same line, but 'lapse' appearing slightly lower by a few pixels. This appeared strange to me that a title signifying a distortion in time was in fact itself distorted! Is this just a coincidence? I think there is more to it than that. It could be the fact

David Stocks

that I have written about some kind of manipulation of time that triggered an event which altered the subheading title in a visual interpretation of the phenomenon. So could this be a sign? Am I being given a clue as to what a time lapse could be?

The following deductions can be made: Time is running on two levels. This mimics a lava flow with the top level of time (the one that we are normally on) flowing slowly, like the crust on the top of the lava flow. The lower level of time flows faster, like the liquid lava below the crust. We experience a time lapse when we occasionally break through the crust to the fast flowing time stream below. The crust must have some elasticity so that when we break through the crust of slow moving time, we actually warp the slow time stream and don't break right through, holding in the faster moving faster time stream until the pull of the upper time stream brings us back to normal time.

These musings didn't keep the voices at bay; they crept deeper inside my consciousness until I couldn't distinguish them from reality. I heard people call my name when they were not addressing me and I would hear friends and relations speak to me when they were not around. This deeply disturbed me; my mind could not distinguish between reality and deception, leaving me to address the dark shadows of my consciousness.

The Celtic Holy Grail Quest

An interesting breakthrough in science has occurred since the writing of this chapter, that of water borne 'Bio metric propulsion systems,' or to put it more precisely a 'Robo Salmon.' The robotic salmon has been designed and engineered by a team from Glasgow University and it resembles a natural salmon in the way it looks and swims, using tail and fin movements to propel it through the water. The salmon is to be used in research, studying the conditions when a salmon decides to use a fish ladder (a series of pools that the salmon leaps up in order to get past a dam). It is fitted with an array of sensors including a water flow meter and more interestingly a camera. Another suggested use is in defence (in the event of a nuclear attack, we would be able to launch a barrage of water borne 'Robo Salmon' - I bet they won't expect that!) Forget Star Wars, we could launch an offshore defence initiative SHOAL (Salmon of Hiroshima Offshore Anti-ballistic Lasers), akin to the Star Wars strategic defence initiative. Our small Island could be surrounded by a large shoal of 'Robo Salmon,' fitted with advanced missile tracking systems and high energy lasers which could be beamed onto incoming missiles, vaporising them before impact. Because of the enormous energy required to generate the killing laser beam a unique 'Nuclear Fission' generator would be built into the salmon.

With all the secrecy that surrounds the 'Robo Salmon,' it is possible to come to all sorts of conjectures as to its true purpose. I believe it has

David Stocks

many possible uses, but in actual fact it was built with one goal in mind, that of locating the 'Salmon of Knowledge.' When you think about it, it all makes sense, what better apparatus is there for such a task? A robotic salmon that looks and swims like a salmon, equipped with an array of sensors capable of detecting the one and only 'Salmon of Knowledge.'

The Celtic Holy Grail Quest

Chapter 26 The appearance and disappearance of Dr Yorkstone

My regular psychiatric doctor was ill for a few months. He was a very good doctor but he was never able to pinpoint my illness. While he was signed off sick he had a replacement, Dr Yorkstone, who was a very amiable old man and must have been at least 75 years old. Talking to him was like talking to a long lost friend. His surgery was a warm oak panelled room lined with books and antique furniture. Dr Yorkstone echoed his surroundings; the timeworn honey coloured wood matched his warm genial features. Whereas most doctors' appointments lasted twenty minutes at the most, when I went to see Dr Yorkstone our sessions went on for well over an hour. He was interested in everything that I said and seemed to understand me better than anyone else could, even me! Initially after our consultation, he recommended an increase in the medication that I was currently on. I left happy that I had not only found a new doctor, but a new friend!

I tried this increase in medication, but after a month or so there was still no improvement. I went back to see Dr Yorkstone for my next appointment. Again we had a long, relaxed and friendly discussion. This time he decided to prescribe a new drug. This was the latest form of a drug that had been around for a while. The symptoms I had been describing to the doctor included racing thoughts, particularly at night. This drug was supposed to calm down such manic symptoms. It is not initially prescribed as it is quite an expensive drug and is known as Valporate Semisodium.

I started taking this drug and quickly noticed an improvement. Although my mind was still overactive especially during the night, my mood had calmed down to an extent that I was able to sleep. With sleep my mood improved and I was able to function more normally. I wasn't able to go back and see Dr Yorkstone immediately as I went on holiday. As soon as I returned from my holiday I was eager to see Dr Yorkstone, but upon making an appointment was disappointed to find that the original doctor was back. I realised with much sadness and trepidation that I would not be able to see Dr Yorkstone again. When I saw my original doctor he was really pleased to see how much progress I had made and referred me to a psychiatric nurse. On meeting the psychiatric nurse I enquired after Dr Yorkstone and whether I could see him again? She replied rather vaguely, 'I'm not sure I know of him and if he was here, then he has probably retired.'

I have nothing but fond memories of Dr Yorkstone; he was such a lovely, likeable old man and it appears that he was sent especially to cure me.

With sleep came dreams and every night I had vivid dreams that assaulted all the senses. In the

The Celtic Holy Grail Quest

morning I could always remember the dreams and some of these I recorded in a dream diary.

Analysing my diary set me to wondering as to the purpose of dreams? Is it to replay passed experiences and learn from them? If you sleep on a problem, when you awake are you better able to deal with it? Are some dreams shared? Do dreams contain messages that you should act on? Are dreams in fact a glimpse into other dimensions where you are living a different life?

These are all questions in need of answers. I have had many strange dreams, as I am sure many people have. Here are a few examples:

I dreamt that I was carrying a monkfish (a fish about a foot to two foot long, with huge wide jaws and hundreds of sharp teeth). Behind the big head the fish had a long stubby triangle of a tail and its jaws were attached to a coat hanger. I carried this coat hanger with the Monkfish attached trying to look casual and inconspicuous as I wondered throughout the duty free shops in an airport. I then had to go through passport control and a security check. I was then asked if I had anything to declare and trying my best to look innocent (hiding the monkfish behind my back) I said I had nothing. The dream then stopped and went back to the beginning, where I tried a different route through the shops, always ending at customs. There must be a moral to this story, the most obvious one being:-

David Stocks

'Don't try to smuggle savage looking fish through customs.'

A more analytical approach would be my lack of self esteem, whereby I feel self-conscious in my job as a fishmonger and try to hide my role from the public.

Another dream I had was that I was trying to contact some friends who live in Montserrat using my landline phone, but was constantly unsuccessful. I decided to contact them using my mobile phone that I was sure had their recent phone number listed and this time managed to get hold of them. When I awoke the next morning my wife told me she had dreamed of phoning our friends in Montserrat using a mobile phone.

This synchronicity in dreams suggests that in the subconscious dream-state we are more in tune psychically and what one dreams the other picks up.

As previously mentioned in this book, the state between waking and sleeping is known as the hypnogogic state and as demonstrated by the dream, it is an altered state of consciousness when our psychic senses are more in tune with our surroundings. By writing much of this book within this state I have been able to view the world with renewed clarity. Like wiping the dust from a dirty window and letting the rays of sun shine through, I am able to perceive things that have been obscured by the psychic pollution of the modern world.

The Celtic Holy Grail Quest

One final experience I would like to relate - I know not if it was a dream or reality - I awoke from a deep sleep soon after moving in to my first house. It was the middle of the night and outside I could hear children singing old fashioned nursery rhymes. Their voices were as clear as bells and the singing went on for a few minutes. Doctors would put this down as lucid dreaming, where you wake but your mind is still experiencing a dream. Everyone at sometime has experienced waking from a dream and temporarily thinking it is real, such is its clarity. This was separate from a dream however; I don't recall the singing while I was asleep and when I woke up I could hear it clearly for a number of minutes. I believe that I experienced some kind of psychic echo that slipped through time and at some time in history there really were children singing outside.

David Stocks

Chapter 27 Energy lines

Autumn closed into winter and dark winter days spread out before me. I retreated into my own dismal cave, my mind shut off from the rest of the world, entering a hibernation period of recluse and solitude. It was a time of rest and regeneration, where my thoughts could wander through old neural pathways trying to break down the mental walls of stress and depression, accessing the contented thoughts that had long since drifted away.

In the house I shared with my wife we had an Inglenook fireplace, in which nested a black iron stove. I would spend many a winter's night staring contentedly into the flames mesmerized by the flickering patterns they made. The flames would have a hypnotic effect upon me and I would soon find myself entering a state of peace. In this state I would occasionally feel myself become detached from my body and be able to drift up with the flames out of the chimney. From here I would begin an astral voyage forever upwards and outwards. I would experience the stars rushing through me, sparking the neurons in my brain and sense the gentle healing power of the cosmos; a feeling of oneness with it all, an understanding that everything was part of a whole and that all the infinite parts of the universe interconnected with one another.

The Celtic Holy Grail Quest

Examining interconnectedness, I perceived a greater understanding of the universal whole. The body has energy lines with key points having been mapped out by our elders for healing. The ancient Chinese developed acupuncture, as far back as 2500 BC. They believed in a dualistic cosmic theory of yin and yang. The yin, the female principle, is passive and dark and is represented by the earth; the yang, the male principle, is active and light and is represented by the heavens. An imbalance of yin and yang results in an obstruction of the vital life force, or chi, in the body. Chi flows through 12 meridians throughout the body and acupuncture is the precise placing of needles over the 12 major meridians and sometimes over a number of specialised minor meridians, in order to bring back the correct balance of yin and yang within the body. Similarly in Hinduism and Buddhism there is an energy field around the body called an aura. The aura is linked to the body by personal energy centres called chakras. Stones, crystals, animals and trees also vibrate with cosmic life-force. The placing of stones and crystals upon vital points on the body can balance the body's chakras and lead to healing.

I believe that the Celts understanding of Mother Earth and of the heavens, have led to the placing of stone monoliths and stone circles at key points on ley lines throughout the world (the Celts had male sky Gods and female earth Gods.) Ley lines are lines of force that are said to traverse the land

and it has been said they are the flight paths of dragons, which may be an ancient Celtic explanation for unexplained phenomenon occurring along these lines. The alignment of these stones has linked them to cosmic energy lines. In effect the ancient people understood something that we do not understand today; that there are universal or even multidimensional energy forces that need balancing, be it with needles, crystals and stones on the body or standing stones and trees on earth. This could also encompass stars, pulsars and black holes on a universal scale. Harmony must be preserved throughout the whole and this is something that modern man has lost touch with. It is only through synchronicity with earth and the stars that healing of this planet can be achieved. If this lost knowledge is not regained then only oblivion awaits mankind.

The practice of Geomancy taps into this ancient wisdom by placing iron rods at key points along ley lines. Let's hope that more research into planetary harmony and Geomancy heals the scars inflicted by modern man.

The Celtic Holy Grail Quest

Chapter 28 The Gamston Triangle

I left work just after ten o'clock on a foggy evening in October. The air was crisp and cold and the ground was slippery with ice. I made my way through Gamston back towards my home. I crossed some fields dimly lit by the little moonlight that seeped through the fog; the frosted blades of grass shimmered silver as they reflected back the light. The fog took on an eerie glow, electrically charged by the night. What phantasms lay suspended in that frozen fusion of moonlight and mist? Ahead lay an alleyway in which the mist had gathered into a dense mass, choking the entrance and rendering the passageway pitch black.

I passed from the silvery night into the alley with some trepidation and as I made my hesitant steps forward I was engulfed in total darkness, consumed by the night. My footsteps echoed from the walls on either side of me, all else was deathly silent. As I strode on I had the inescapable feeling that I was being swallowed up by a black hole where forces of light lay dormant and everything was dragged down into its deep dark depths. What demons lay in wait for me within its inky black folds? My mind and spirit were being eaten from within by fear. The darkness outside lay seed to my dark fears inside. I sensed the walls of the alley pressing in on me, hidden demons reaching out to grab me. If I didn't escape this passage, I would be crushed in their evil grip. I moved into a

David Stocks

run, the fog now so dense that it felt like I was pushing my way through treacle. Disorientated I bounced off the walls in my blind panic to free myself of the dark throat of the alley. The fog had become so dense it was sticking to my lungs, making breathing difficult, until gasping for breath I staggered out of the passage and was born into a new world.

The air was crisp and clear and I drank in its freshness, my lungs heaving with the exertion. Ahead of me lay the village green, a shimmering silver triangle lit by the moonlight. I was drawn towards this mystical oasis, a sparkling diamond in a fog strewn desert. I entered the green by a small wooden gate, a gateway to another dimension, a transitory meeting place of two worlds. Time rolled backwards, the mist swirled round the green in a vortex as the wheel of time spun in reverse, back to an age long forgotten. I staggered and fell backwards. Lying on my back I looked up at the moon, which hung clear and bright in the night sky. The mist spun in a funnel down from it, leaving me on my island of calm of Gamston village green.

Electricity charged the air and blue lightning shot up and down the vortex as it continued to gather speed. The storm gathered in momentum and intensity until all at once it stopped. The silence was deafening, but something had changed. Leaves fell like snowflakes upon the ground. All around me stood wooden posts joined at the top

The Celtic Holy Grail Quest

by oak lintels. My head rested against something rough and hard. Looking up I discovered that my resting place was a huge oak tree. What startled me more was the man standing opposite me in the shadow of the tree. He wore rough brown and green hemp trousers and a tunic. He stood a good seven feet tall and rested one hand on a stout stave, but his most startling feature was his face. This was as old as time and entirely made up of foliage, oak leaves and vines that replaced normal facial features. He could only be the Green Man and as such should be venerated.

I stood in awe of this creature of myth and legend and gazed transfixed into his acorn like eyes. Who am I to behold such a being, nature's messenger to her earthen brethren? How mighty he stood, bearing his solid oaken features and I realised that he was ancient, yet just a child of the tree behind me. And then he spoke in both riddle and rhyme, a message he gave me as old as time. In a language long forgotten, I listened to his words, which I understood despite the ancient verse.

And so in a creaking voice both knotted and gnarled he spoke these words, which only I heard.

> When the next lunar cycle,
> Reaches its zenith,
> Nature's disciple,
> Go forthwith,
> To the ground of the dead,
> High on a hilltop,

David Stocks

Past the guardian's head,
With a cavernous backdrop
Into the fiery depths,
You must travel,
Along treacherous paths,
A maze unravel,
To the crystal cave,
And the pool of souls,
Across which you must brave,
To achieve all your goals.

Then with these words he strode away. I was suddenly overcome with exhaustion and resting my head against the trunk of the ancient oak I fell asleep.

I dreamt of giant black hounds with fiery eyes that pierced my soul and then attempted to rip it from my body. My soul appeared as a flickering blue light that ran up and down my spine and through my skull. The hounds would bite the end of this thread as it came out of my skull and attempt to wrench it from me. They did not succeed, however, as it was woven into my spine in the form of a Celtic knot and it stretched from my skull but did not release.

I awoke refreshed despite my uncomfortable dreams and felt green sap rising through my veins. The tree on which I had been resting had gone. Across the way lay a pole; it was a broken off branch of a tree, slender and strong. It was unusually straight and had fresh sap oozing from

The Celtic Holy Grail Quest

it. I looked around but could not see from which tree it had broken. The fog had cleared from around the green and I made my way back out through the gate and across the courtyard to my house, taking the pole with me.

Logic dictates that my Celtic research and knowledge of the Green Man led to a lucid dream in which the Green Man appeared. But dreams are subtle things and know no boundaries. My mind may have generated the experience with the Green Man based on prior knowledge, or it may have been a call from the past, a guiding hand on my quest.

Wide awake now, I spent the rest of the night searching books on the history of Nottingham, trying to find any Celtic connections that it may have, and eventually stumbling across an old name for it, 'Tigguocobauc.'

Further research on the internet the next day uncovered the translation for it; it was an early Celtic name for Nottingham: 'Tigguocobauc' or 'City of Caves.'

David Stocks

Chapter 29 The path of the dead

So what were these caves and where might they lie? I knew Nottingham was littered with caves but where should I start? I began my search at Nottingham Castle where I knew there were caves, the most famous of these being Mortimer's Hole. I took a tour down Mortimer's Hole which was an old passageway leading to a waterway below.

I went with my father and we were the only two people to turn up for the tour that day. Our tour guide refused to take our money as a tour could not officially be run with less than three people. Two people, therefore, obviously didn't constitute a tour! I thought about mentioning my two little friends on my shoulders, but thought better of it. He did however take us, for he was an enthusiast and enjoyed showing us the long forgotten pathways of Nottingham and beguiling us with historic tales of intrigue and drama from times long gone by.

Before descending into the depths of Mortimer's Hole, our enthusiastic guide took us on a tour of the grounds of Nottingham Castle. He took great delight in regaling us with historic moments in the castle's history, with tales of intrigue and war, since the castle's inception. The man was a veritable history book of facts and figures. My father and I just nodded sagely as our guide, not

The Celtic Holy Grail Quest

needing any encouragement, pointed out scenes of great battles from the vantage point of Castle Rock.

It was with some reluctance that he eventually left his foot soldiers to continue the siege of Nottingham Castle, while he frogmarched us to the passage that was Mortimer's Hole. It had been carved out of sandstone centuries ago as a way of transporting goods up to the castle.

Mortimer's Hole acquired its name after the successful abduction of Edward III by Roger Mortimer, Earl of March. Mortimer was said to have used the tunnel as a way of sneaking into the castle, where his group surprised and killed the guards and abducted Edward III. Other accounts say that he took a different passage using passwords to get through a postern gate and then returning via Mortimer's Hole.

The passageway curved spectacularly in the rock with red striations running throughout, like the most glorious sunset on weathered clay hills. It was while we were being guided around the cave, that other caves at a cemetery were mentioned. These were located in the aptly named 'Rock Cemetery,' at the top of Mansfield Road. This cemetery was renowned for its caves and had a commanding hilltop location.

We emerged from Mortimer's Hole at the bottom of Castle Rock and left our tour guide to rally his

David Stocks

troops. We made our way to the famous 'Trip to Jerusalem,' the oldest inn in England. This pub is one of my favourite pubs anywhere and it is itself partly made up of caves. When the knights were on the crusades to the Holy Land, they used to stop at this inn for refreshments, hence the name 'Trip to Jerusalem.' These very knights may have been the same ones who originally quested for the Holy Grail at the site of the ancient temple of Solomon. If this was the favourite watering hole of the original Grail knights, then it would certainly do for my father and me. We strode in to the bar and ordered a couple of pints of holy water.

We sat in the dark recesses of one of the inn's caves, supping our ale and discussing knights, the Grail and all things holy. We got on to the topic of the old model ship that hung from the ceiling. It has hung there for no-one knows how long, gathering the dust of centuries, as it sailed through the seas of time. It is well known to be a 'cursed galleon' and anyone who dares to touch it and move it is deemed to be cursed. I felt like I had stepped into a time capsule, to a world in which valiant knights trod and cursed galleons sailed. In more recent times the inn has been refurbished, still maintaining its original integrity and character, but the Galleon has been moved. By whom I don't know, but whoever that brave soul was I can only hope that they have not succumbed to the ancient curse.

'Ye Olde Trip to Jerusalem' is certainly a place to

The Celtic Holy Grail Quest

go if you want atmosphere and I enjoyed a particularly good evening there once on a story tellers' night. Once a month, story tellers gather at the Trip to Jerusalem and tell tales of mystery, intrigue and romance. One particular gathering had as its theme vampires, this being the one that my wife and I attended.

We sat sipping blood red wine, while unholy tales of vampires biting the delicate white flesh of virgins' necks and draining them of blood were spun. Candles flickered in recesses, shadows reached across the walls of the cave and fell on the unsuspecting. The tension grew as ever more chilling tails were regaled, reaching a climax when the Master Story Teller himself took centre stage. Everyone huddled around him as he told us a spine tingling tale of a lone man wandering the streets of upper Nottingham at night. Coincidently he ventured into the very cemetery that the guide had told my father and I about, the one riddled with caves. He wove a tail of dread and fear, of things unholy wandering the hallowed ground of this old cemetery, through broken tombstones and fallen angels. In this most lonesome place one poor individual accidentally strayed and soon became lost, his fear building as he rounded shattered tombs from which skeletal hands protruded. His fears were finally realised when towards him drifted a cloaked figure gliding on a carpet of mist through that sacred ground. All was silent in the dark interior of the cave in the back of the pub. The Master Story Teller drew on the

David Stocks

suspense and our insides churned in turmoil ... the cloaked figure slowly turned round and revealed his face, shadowed by the high collar of the cloak he was wearing, to the fearful lost individual. It was the moment of dread, everyone was quiet ... it was a face well known, a face that has sent many a pure maiden weak at the knees ... it was the face of Elvis Presley.

The rest of the story became ever more comical; I cannot recall the entire tale but it involved anoraks and a shared interest in train spotting.

Having set the ambient scene for the graveyard, I shall return to the main thread of the story.

With the information that I had gathered so far I could solve the first part of the riddle, as posed by the Green Man:

> When the next lunar cycle,
> Reaches its zenith,
> (The next full moon)
> Nature's disciple,
> Go forthwith,
> (Head out with the nature's evergreen staff)
> To the ground of the dead,
> High on a hilltop,
> (Journey to Rock Cemetery).

The secrets held within the rest of the riddle still alluded me. So when was the next full moon? I checked in my diary and felt a cold hand clutch at

The Celtic Holy Grail Quest

my soul for it was soon, October 17th; not long before the passing of the year, a time when spirits wander the earth, the nearest full moon to Halloween.

Halloween originated as the Celtic festival of Samhain. It marked the end of an old year and the beginning of a new one. It was a time when fearsome beasts and monsters walked the earth, a time when the gateways to the otherworld were open and spirits roamed terra-firma. If ever there was a time to step through the fabric of the real world and walk the path of the dead to the underworld, then the full moon closest to Samhain was the appropriate time.

I dreamt that night of angels. I walked through corridors of them, each one smiling serenely and pointing the way ahead. I would follow their lead but always end up back at the place from whence I started.

I needed to do some more research on Samhain, but where did I start? I then remembered the old shopkeeper in Lincoln. I took out his card, which I kept in my wallet and looked at it:

   Mr A. Chronostella
   Antiquarian, purveyor of books,
   Maps and Curiosities,
   Both ancient and old.

I dialled the number on the back of the card and

David Stocks

after a few short rings I got an answer.

'Mr Chronostella here, how can I help?' he answered in a mellow timbered voice, with all the subtleties of a 20 year old whisky.
'Hi, I don't know if you remember me?' The shopkeeper interrupted me and said, 'Of course I do, you're the gentleman on the trail of the Celtic Holy Grail.' 'Yes, that's right, I was wondering if you could help me further with this quest?'

I went on to explain where my research had led me and my interest in the full moon approaching the Celtic festival of Samhain.

'Ah, I see where you are heading; it would appear to me that you are being dream guided. This can be a good or bad thing depending on which spirits are leading you. Trust your instincts, they should see you through. As for Samhain, this is where the real world and the spirit world intertwine and it is possible as a mortal to enter the spirit world if the correct actions are taken. The full moon nearest this event is an auspicious time when nature brings the material and immaterial into close proximity to each other where boundaries may be crossed.'

'Do you believe it is possible to find the otherworld if I enter this cemetery and venture down into the cavernous depths at this time?' I asked.

'Oh, during the fluxing of the year anything is

The Celtic Holy Grail Quest

possible and it may well be that you will reach your goal, but I warn you that you will be severely tested in mind body and spirit. Light a lamp, this will attract friendly spirits to you and guide them home,' the shopkeeper replied.

'Do you have any idea as to what form the tests will take?' I enquired.
' The tests will be on three levels:-
Firstly: the mind. Your worst fears will be visited upon you, those from the innermost darkest depths of your mind that you keep locked away. The mind's demons will become real and the real surreal. There is only one way that these demons can be banished and that is by confronting them directly and facing your fears.
Secondly, the body: The physical test will be just as arduous as the mental one. You will have to make your way through an underworld labyrinth; of what form this will take I can only speculate, but great demands will be put on your physical body.
Thirdly, the spirit: This is the least recognised human attribute in modern man, something lost to man with the rise of culture and technology. In order to attain the Grail you must become one with your spiritual side.'

I thanked him for the advice and he in turn wished me good luck on my quest. His parting words to me were: 'Find yourself.'

And so I waited for October 17th, the full moon on the cusp of Halloween, Samhain and the contents

David Stocks

of my dreams.

The Celtic Holy Grail Quest

Chapter 30 Gypsies, Bombs and Pantomime Cows

Before the coming of the full moon and Samhain, I changed jobs and became a Barista at a coffee shop, just off the Old Market Square in Nottingham. This I found a rewarding job as I worked with many different personalities and lots of young and exiting people. Of great help and importance to my recovery from depression and its associated mental traumas, was contact with people.
Through interactions with others I was able to escape the clutches of depression; the distraction helped but most of all camaraderie. By being amongst people I did not cut myself off from society and I found within that innate human quality for bonding and friendship.
Depression is at its worst when one is alone. At times - and there have been many in my case - social contact is daunting. Being of a naturally shy disposition I often feel intimidated by the presence of other people, to such an extent that I sometimes can't bear to be touched. All I can say is keep your own private space in times of great stress and anxiety, but whenever possible open yourself up to contact with other people. I don't say let everyone know if you suffer from depression, but most people are very helpful if you let your worries be known - it is part of human nature. You can usually tell if it is not wise to reveal a so called mental illness and I personally

David Stocks

believe depression can help build a more beautiful person inside.

The coffee shop was a new one in a highly respected chain of coffee shops. Although the coffee shops are now owned by a parent company, it maintains its original ethos and all new employees go to its headquarters in London for training. It being a new team, we all went together for our training, thus making it a team building exercise as well. And so it was that we arrived at the place where the chain of coffee shops originated, the home of Costa Coffee.

As I write this, I sip from a cup of Italian roasted coffee, its aroma percolating through the house and reminding me of my days at Costa. Note: I am drinking Italian roasted coffee, for it is Italians who have refined the art of coffee making and excel in all aspects of the coffee process from plantation to cup. To be Italian is to love coffee. It is therefore appropriate that one of Britain's leading chains of coffee shops was founded by Italians.

I was honest with my manager regarding my history of depression, but proved myself on the shop floor by not just serving coffee, but listening to and joking with the customers. He was open minded and forward thinking, wanting more than just a team for the new coffee shop, but one that combines service with character. The team that he built had no shortage of those!

When you join Costa you join a family and learn to respect its family values. I liken it to the Italian Mafia that takes pride in operating as one big family, but without the criminal associations of

The Celtic Holy Grail Quest

which the Mafia is renowned. To this purpose I nicknamed the Costa, 'Costa Nostra' after the Sicilian Mafia, Cosa Nostra. Gino, Costa's master roaster, is the father figure of the Costa family. The headquarters is based by a railway in the east end of London and the coffee beans are stored under railway arches, the perfect conditions for keeping the beans. The beans are then slow roasted in large vats to give the perfect flavour. When Gino inspects the roaster, the workers are said to whistle the Godfather tune, for Gino is the Godfather of the Costa Nostra.

The bronze award induction training only lasts a day, but during that time the core principles of producing the perfect cup of coffee are instilled into you. I learnt more in that day than I ever have in the numerous training courses I have attended before or since. I have been trained in project management, sales, marketing and countless computer technologies, but none rewarded me with more wisdom than the Costa induction course. From this I learnt the core values of customer service, attention to detail, pride in my product and accepting only the highest standards of delivery.

Not one for doing things by halves, our manager opened the new Costa coffee shop on Nottingham Market Square in style. When I say style, it was not so much style as attention grabbing. Enter the pantomime cow! What on earth has a pantomime cow got to do with the opening of a coffee shop? Not a lot actually, but it achieved its aim; the new Costa opening did not go unnoticed. I achieved

David Stocks

my moment of fame; I can safely say that I am the only person to ever have marched across the Old Market Square in the centre of Nottingham as the rear end of a pantomime cow. By choice, this is not the preferential end of the cow, but through lack of inhibitions and other suitable volunteers, I took on the role. The advertising stunt was to promote a prize being given out by Costa, of winning a cow which could be donated to a needy country. The press were there and I have many famous shots, standing in the market square as the rear end of Daisy the cow.

From these dubious foundations I learnt the trade, coming out of myself and building a repartee with both the customers and my colleagues. I was serving coffee, Italian style, with flair. I was helped by my management and in particular an Italian called Francesco. He was a real character, always with a smile, but prone to an Italian temperament.

Together Francesco and I formed a dynamic Anglo-Italian duo and would always be having a laugh and joking with each other. Francesco was second to none on the coffee machine and he would complain in Italian if we weren't calling the orders to him. To which I would react by putting on my best Italian accent and shouting loudly across the bar in mock Italian, comments of the following ilk: 'Doppio espressio, mucho creamio, mucho mucho choclatio!' - explaining to the customers that our little Sardinian friend would only take

The Celtic Holy Grail Quest

orders in Italian, but luckily I could speak it fluently.
This would cause a tirade of Italian muttering and cursing from Francesco.

On another occasion, Francesco, impatient to get a customer's order would start bypassing me (even though it was my job to take orders at the till) by asking the customers directly for their orders. Francesco being Italian was naturally the best at making coffee and so was stationed at the coffee machine. After much arguing we resolved the issue by Francesco standing behind me and calling out the orders, while I mouthed what he was saying silently!

On occasions it was necessary to leave the coffee shop on errands to get milk or pay money into the bank. It was on one such errand that I left the coffee shop and made my way across the square. As I strode across the Old Market Square I felt like an Italian priest in my black vestments and the long black apron of my coffee shop uniform flapping in the wind.

History was stripped away and I found myself mysteriously alone in the square, despite it being one of the busiest times of the year in Nottingham. It was the first Wednesday in October, the start of the Goose Fair.

Out through the mists of time came an old gypsy woman. She wore a patchwork shawl and

David Stocks

burgundy headscarf.

'Sprig of heather for luck, me love?' she asked. Being superstitious and in need of some luck, I bought a sprig from her and she smiled then whispered in my ear, 'Twice shall ye visit the realm of the dead and twice shall ye be reborn. Thy mind's demons will linger, burning with a fever and then no more. Out of despair's own ashes shall rise hope and fulfilment.'

And then she was a gone, a faint whisper on the winds of time, back when Goose Fair was originally held on the Old Market Square.

I felt a chill pass through me and was at a loss as to the meaning of her words, but time was to reveal all to me.

One more incident regarding the Old Market square is worth retelling.

I was out on the town one night when the whole of the area surrounding the market square was cordoned off. All the bars and pubs were evacuated, all the premises vacated. The police took control.

It was not until the next day that I discovered the cause of this exodus. On returning to work at Costa I found the door had been broken away from its hinges. On further enquiry, I was told a suspect package had been found. This was at a

The Celtic Holy Grail Quest

time of heightened security; there had just been bombings in London.

The full story unravelled itself to me. One of the baristas had found an unattended bag within the cafe. It was quite a large bag and contained an unmarked box. No-one turned up to retrieve it and the police were called in. Unable to identify the contents of the box, the Old Market Square was evacuated and the bomb disposal team took over. A robotic device was then sent in to the shop, breaking open the door to gain access. It proceeded to perform a controlled explosion. Examination of the debris later revealed that Nottingham was now safe from the dangers of a well distributed garden table.

David Stocks

Chapter 31 Full moon floating in a blood red sky

I made my pilgrimage to Rock Cemetery on October 17th just as the sun was setting. I stood at the entrance, iron gates swung wide, with my green staff in one hand and flickering lantern in the other. With the hood up on my coat, I looked every part the Celtic disciple. The air was crisp and clear and the sun glowed vibrantly as it sank on the horizon. I made my way into the cemetery along an avenue of tombstones, with statues of angels perched serenely on their tops silhouetted against the setting sun.

As the sun made its exit, the sky glowed blood red and the full moon could be seen floating in a sea of blood with clouds like waves washing against its surface. The old year was burning out and the new year igniting on this special night.

The path I was following was like a main artery through the graveyard pumping red with the light of the sunset. I continued along this vein in search of its ghostly heart. I descended on a path, cut through the rocks with graves hewn out of sandstone on either side of me. The ornamentation on some of the graves was quite elaborate, with tombs carved out of rock to resemble houses complete with gabled roofs. Some graves had what looked like Masonic symbols carved on them and Celtic crosses were

The Celtic Holy Grail Quest

in abundance - a positive omen.

The evening became distinctly chilly as the red glow faded from the sky and the silver blue light of twilight diffused into the night sky. Everything took on sinister connotations. Age and decay bore down on the lower reaches of the graveyard. Gravestones stood either broken or leaning to one side, as if their skeletal inhabitants were trying to force their way out of their earthen graves. Roots and branches clawed at me from the rocky walls. Deep holes beckoned me from the sides of the path. One false step would send me careening down helpless into a bottomless chasm. I felt the urge to turn back from this haunting path to the unknown and return to higher planes. My mind was starting to play tricks on me; images of demons lurked in the shadows hidden behind gravestones in the dark depths of the tombs. I hardened my resolve, quickened my pace and marched resolutely onwards.

Before the onset of the evening's quest, I had left the kitchen table set with a black cloth, a candle and one place setting. On this setting I had placed a hearty meal; this was a meal for the dead, an offering to the spirits to give them sustenance in the afterlife. I hoped these spirits would protect me on this evening's journey, but as I descended I could only sense evil. Still I had to cling on to the hope that they would offer some protection.

The path ended abruptly at a sandstone wall. I

cast my gaze downwards over the wall and stared into a huge rock hewn arena, hell's own pit. I stood there transfixed by this forum, out of which a high pitched keening wail reverberated, echoing off its walls. Frozen to the spot, my heart skipped a beat and a cold shiver shot down my spine. It was a jagged cry of sorrow and grief, a grim portent of death, for it was the cry of a banshee, the harbinger of death. Every muscle in my body wanted to turn and run, flee the danger, the imminent death that surely awaited me. Still I couldn't move, I had to fight the fear, for in fear lies despair and in despair resides my own personal hell. I geared myself up to confront my demons and fought against the urge to flee them. This demon was all too real however, not a demon of the mind, or was it? I was beginning to lose focus but held my resolve and turning I followed a broad ramp spiralling down into hell's arena.

The chilling cry reverberated louder still as I made my descent, crashing over me in waves of fear, a viscous sea of noise in which I swam, trying to avoid drowning in its terrifying depths. Ancient sandstone walls towered over me and I was consumed by paranoid thoughts that they were not there as external defences but had a more sinister purpose, that of containment, to keep something in, but what? I sensed a distinctly malevolent presence lying within this dark compound. Rounding the final bend I finished my unholy descent, my foot striking a gravestone embedded in the arena floor. It formed a perfect

The Celtic Holy Grail Quest

circle and seemed to reflect the moon above. I could see that it had been excavated for this very purpose, it was a mirror to capture the image of the full moon. Silvery blue light spread out across the floor, carpeted in gravestones and as I made my way across I was literally walking the path of the dead.

All around the arena were caves out of which mist started to issue forth: the breath of the dead. Into this mist I ventured towards the cavernous mouth of the largest of these openings. Wind snaked throughout the hidden passages of the arena, generating the soulful wail of the banshee, which transformed it in a far deeper, bloodcurdling howl of the devil's own hound. What awaited me as I entered the deepest darkest chamber, the chamber of horrors, the theatre of fear; a place where your darkest nightmares come out to play and feast on your mind, soul and body?

In my feverish mind, giant jaws gaped open before me. Doormath the hellhound, guardian of the underworld, had come to meet me. To enter the underworld I must pass Doormath. Blindly and irrationally I stumbled through those jaws, consumed in mist: the breath of the underworld.

Somewhere in my rational mind I knew that nature was playing tricks on me and this was all the conjuring of my imagination, but at the same time I felt in touch with the mystical world of the Celtic otherworld and was voyaging much in the same

David Stocks

way as the ancient Celtic shamans did eons ago. Conjurations of the mind? Imagination? Imagination left unchecked brings the underworld closer. A child is wiser than its parents. The preconditioning of human nature as dictated by our elders is a false cloak. In a child's innocence it sees things that modern man refuses to accept.

I stumbled upon a hard earthen floor. Dazed, I held the lantern above me and cast its light back from whence I came. Silver shafts of light shimmered in the mist gushing past me through the aperture of the cave. I could now make out the twisted, pointed iron bars that I had previously distinguished as Doormath's jaws; an ancient myth transformed into an urban myth, jagged blood stained teeth formed from ferrous rusted iron bars.

In my hand I still held the staff I had found on Gamston Green, still green with sap, symbolising life in the otherworld, my lantern a guide for lost spirits. Holding my beacon of light aloft I rose to my feet, scattering discarded needles left by hapless junkies who had undertaken trips of their own (although of a much more hazardous nature to their health). I ventured into the maze of tunnels that stretched beneath the long since decayed bodies of the cemetery's inhabitants.

I could feel the spirits of the past, present and future calling me into their domain. The staff I held kept me both in the real world and the surreal otherworld at the same time. Its textured bark bit

The Celtic Holy Grail Quest

into my hand, reminding me of reality and the vitality of its sap connected me with nature and the spirits of the underworld.

I wandered the corridors of the dead letting instinct guide me through the myriad of turnings I took. The rough hewn passages gave forth demonic shapes transmogrified from simple rocky outcrops to diabolic fantasies. Dark shadows stretched inky black fingers out towards me. Hidden recesses whispered in the draughty chambers of unimagined horrors. Cold wet mist clung in tendrils to my skin and formed moist cobwebs in my hair, like ectoplasm from the spirits of the dead, and dripped cold tears down my forehead.

I journeyed on until exhaustion took its toll. Totally disorientated I found myself in a circular chamber sunken in the middle, in which mist spiralled lazily around. I gazed into its whirling depths and was mesmerized by the silvery layers spinning round interlacing in and out in an eternal Celtic knot. Transfixed I stepped into this natural phenomenon and into the supernatural world of Celtic spirits. I was in a labyrinth of tunnels and caves deep under a cemetery, in a vortex of mist spiralling all around me. I lost myself in its slippery patterns and felt distant childhood memories calling me. I recalled times of adventure, discovering hidden pathways through woods and seeing demons hiding in trees and thickets. I remembered the magic of summer meadows where fairies danced under willow trees by laughing babbling brooks and antarctic journeys through the snowy wilderness of a winter garden, building snowmen

David Stocks

and talking to Eskimos. I regressed and progressed. I spent an indeterminate amount of time, for time had no meaning in this place, transfixed by the silvery tapestry of childhood memories swirling around me. I eventually emerged from the whirlpool of mist and stepped out, reborn with the fresh imagination of a child. Once again I understood the importance of imagination; it is not just a childhood fantasy but a creative process that can lead you into a greater understanding of veil cast over reality. I looked back at the maelstrom of mist and saw in it the legendary cauldron of the Celtic underworld, a cauldron that had gifted me with the wisdom and knowledge of the ancients and of the very young.

Lost upon a Celtic shore I cast myself adrift in the currents that circulated the caverns within and followed their flow, that of the wind, back out of the tunnels and strode out of the Celtic underworld. Despite the arduous journey through caverns untold I felt refreshed and invigorated by my night's ordeals.

The Celtic Holy Grail Quest

Chapter 32 Conan the Librarian and the Lost Library of Bingham

During the winter months I paid regular visits to the gym. Not being a patient person and having a dislike of aerobic activity, I took to doing weights. Exercise, as previously mentioned, gives the body a boost and helps relieve some of the symptoms of depression. The regular exercise, while not turning me into a muscle-bound hulk, did present a more imposing exterior.

After many unsuccessful attempts I secured myself a position as an Assistant Librarian. It was a part-time job and I did it alongside my work at the coffee shop. I did not fit the classical stereotype of a librarian however. I wore no spectacles on a chain around my neck and I did not have the intellectual, scholarly look. In fact with my more robust physique, I was more a semblance of Conan the Librarian. As with all great warrior librarians I was posted to a remote outpost to a library in the small market town of Bingham. I refer to it as 'the lost library of Bingham,' as people who end up there are usually lost and on route to another place entirely.

As you are reading this book you may feel that it is not extraordinary that I should seek employment in a library. To most however, the accepted opinion of a librarian is that of a nerd. It is definitely not a cool job! How many great librarians are known to

David Stocks

history? Hence I created my 'Conan the Librarian' image and the phrase 'The pen is mightier than the sword. If that doesn't work, then throw books at them.'

Having built up my mighty librarian image I will now poor cold water on the raging librarian you have in mind. For the most part I stepped back from conflict with troublemakers within the library. Another image I wish to quell is the age old idea of the silent library. Libraries are up to date, they have computers with internet access and therefore they have kids. Kids make noise, lots of it, and while most of the time this can be kept to a certain level, the library is not the tranquil place of study it once was, in fact far from it. In order not to totally destroy your perception of a raging librarian, I have been known at times to storm across the library and send known troublemakers outside. All with just one word, 'OUT!' said in such a way that there was no doubt as to the outcome. The rest of the time I was placid.

Of course the library was a great place to further my Celtic research and pursue my quest for the Grail. Without the usual restrictions on book withdrawals, I soon had amassed a sizeable library of my own.

Having gained excellent customer service skills I endeavoured to satisfy customers' requirements. My concentration however was poor that turned out to be a result of the medication I was on,

The Celtic Holy Grail Quest

which I will discuss later on in this book. Because I concentrated on customer service to such a high standard, it was considered I was neglecting other tasks and because of my poor concentration I was not considered to be fully up to speed. This did my self esteem no good at all. One thing that is easily lost through depression is self esteem and once lost is very hard to regain. I urge all employers to take care of their staff's self esteem, it is a very valuable asset to everyone. I don't blame my employers for my loss of self esteem, circumstances dictated the course I was on. I only ask that people take into account the importance of self image and help those who are in doubt regarding their worth.

I spent more time on the Internet, constantly amazed how it had evolved over the years and marvelling at the fact that one could go on to the Internet any time, day or night and be in contact with people all over the world. By communicating electronically, a whole new community had been born with the rise of the Internet. Mobile phones, now commonplace, put people in touch practically anywhere in the world. Faster travel by planes, trains and cars was effectively reducing the distance between people. All these things have brought together one global community; the world is now a small world and getting smaller all the time.

As population increases to gargantuan proportions, the ability for earth to support

David Stocks

mankind diminishes. Where do we go from here? It is time for governments to conserve our resources and use their wealth to heal an ailing planet? Unfortunately money is a dictating factor in the hands of people able to progress and regenerate our planet. The most effective way of tackling this issue is for governments to agree on ways of rewarding investment in the planet's future. Only then will money be spent wisely and reconciliation with the planet be made. We can no longer be blind to the effects of rapidly increasing population and ever dwindling resources. It may be that we have to look to colonising new planets, to ease the burden on our own. Massive technological advances are required if this is ever to happen, but who knows, maybe the technology is already out there and has yet to be harnessed?

Is the pen mightier than the sword? I have written these words with such hope and know thousands of people have done so before me. I am not a tree hugger, I believe a more constructive way of reaching a mass audience is through words. I am humble and speak not as a great scholar or scientist, I speak as a human being and what it is to be a true human being. I am nobody special, which is the way I want to be seen, for there are millions of people like me out there who believe in what I believe. If you are reading this then take up your pen, write of deeds yet to be done, of saving the planet and all mankind.

The Celtic Holy Grail Quest

Chapter 33 Dire straits and the search for Atlantis

A recurring theme throughout my research for this book is the legend of Atlantis. Through my collection of books and wanderings along the electronic byways of the Internet, I have stumbled upon many a reference to Atlantis.
I was indeed in a state of dire straits again through the dark period of year winter brings. To keep myself afloat I set a course for Atlantis, both in the historical and metaphorical sense. Reference to Atlantis is first made by Plato in his dialogues Timaeus, its location being described as:-
'And there was an island situated in front of the straits which are by you called the Pillars of Heracles.'
These straits I likened to my dire straits, through which I had to pass in order to reach my own personal Atlantis.
The dialogues concerning Atlantis are solely the account of Critias in the Timaeus dialogues. In it he claims the description of ancient Athens and Atlantis are derived from a visit by Athenian Lawgiver Solon to Egypt in the 6th Century BC. Solon is regaled the tale of ancient Athens and Atlantis. The Egyptian priest Sais reads the story to him, recorded on papyri in Egyptian Hieroglyphs. In the dialogues Atlantis is portrayed as such:
'Now in this island of Atlantis there was a great and wonderful empire which had rule over the

whole island and several others, and over parts of the continent, and, furthermore, the men of Atlantis had subjected the parts of Libya within the columns of Heracles as far as Egypt, and of Europe as far as Tyrrhenia.'

Many future works of fiction have since been based on the Atlantis legend. Another recurring theme in my research is that of the founder of modern scientific method, Francis Bacon. Independently researching Atlantis and Francis Bacon I came upon the same piece of work, 'The New Atlantis.' This is a fictional novel by Francis Bacon on a utopian society, depicting a mythical land called Bensalem. In this land scientific method and experimentation are rewarded. In a college called Salomen's House, Bacon's own style of scientific method is used to tame nature and better mankind.

The famous phrase 'Knowledge is power,' was coined by him. He had powerful friends in his lifetime, including that of King James I, so maybe his pursuit of scientific knowledge did give him power.

There was more than one famous Francis Bacon and he was a descendent of the Elizabethan Francis Bacon just mentioned. I am pursuing a train of thought, the references to Francis Bacon being the path that I am now blindly following. The outcome of this chapter is unknown to me but bear with me on this voyage, for Atlantis is my destination and both famous Francis Bacon incarnations are stepping stones along the way.

The Celtic Holy Grail Quest

So who is this other Francis Bacon? For those who need an introduction, he was a famous figurative painter of the 20th Century.
He painted dark and surreal imagery that is a style I can particularly relate to, the devil's palette applied to the dark canvas of my mind. A misconception of the dark images that so called mentally ill people conjure up is that it is unhealthy, not good for you. This is not the case. To experience a truly dark image is like sipping a vintage wine. One sip and you are seduced by its effects and want to sample more of the subtleties contained therein. A dark image is full of secrets waiting to be discovered and as you sip from that cloaked vessel, watch a cloud pass over the moon and taste the essence of the night. Darkness does not have to be sad, enjoy it as an experience. Without darkness there would be no light; for without darkness there is nothing with which to compare light.

Darkness is but one aspect of life. I like to explore as many facets of life (within reason) that I can. One of the ways I find of breaking out of melancholy is to keep variety in my life. To me variety is the spice of life and I strongly believe if efforts are made to bring variety into your life, then you will reap the rewards. Change can cause many people undue stress, I being a prime example. But I am finding that if I let go and just go with the flow, change that at first seems bad is not such a big problem. Through being able to follow the flow of life more, I have been a lot more content.

I am still on the track of Francis Bacon and following it to wherever it leads me. The 20th century Francis Bacon painted a picture that I have been particularly drawn to. This picture is his study of another famous painting by Diego Velazquez of Pope Innocent X in 1650. He became obsessed by the painting and his interpretation shows a haunting image of the Pope sat on a throne screaming. It is vivid and grabs your attention. Francis Bacon picked up on the not so innocent crafty look of the Pope, as portrayed by Velazquez and turned it into a scream. Prior to becoming Pope, Pope Innocent X was appointed nuncio in Madrid where he may have had the last say. In an interesting quirk of fate Francis Bacon travelled to Madrid in April 1992 where he died of a heart attack; Velazquez died in the same city in 1660.

From Plato's dialogues I have stumbled into the world of art, but am I on the right course for Atlantis? The question is rhetorical, for art is a voyage of discovery itself and fully understanding a work of art is akin to unravelling the Grail mystery. To miss a glance at the world of art, is to miss an opportunity. But as this chapter unfolds, I glimpse Atlantis once again.

I am drawn to Atlantis on a circuitous route, via Picasso's cubist version of the Velazquez painting,

The Celtic Holy Grail Quest

'Las Meninas.' Everyone's perception of art is different and many do not like the more modern forms of painting. To me Picasso's version of Las Meninas is striking in its use of black and white and cubist dimensions. I will not try to dictate art to the reader, for art is a very personal thing and I am a not an expert in the field by any means. The link I finally make to Atlantis is through another medium, that of poetry and a poem called Atlantis written by Miguel Ajeno. This I discovered when looking into Picasso's art. Another poem by Ajeno was found accompanied by art that is very reminiscent of Picasso and formed an introduction to Ajeno's poems.

Miguel Ajeno was an enigmatic figure, a forgotten poet who lived through troubled times in Columbia. His was a voice destined to be heard by few, but could have been a powerful poet of 20th Century Latin America. Only a few poems of his have survived today as a result of external pressures and his beliefs. These poems I have read and are treasured fragments of a man that will last within me forever. In his poem, Atlantis, I see a Columbia before the Conquistadors and all the troubled times that followed. He makes the jungles weep at civilisations lost, nobler than ones that followed. Perhaps Columbia did contain mythical, utopian places, where Atlantis wasn't a dream? The mythical city of El Dorado was once sought there.

David Stocks

With Atlantis back in sight I follow this lead to the Aztec and Myan civilizations that once existed in Central America. Some of the famous cities of these civilizations had massive pyramids. Pyramids of course are famous in Egypt. Many standing stones have been discovered forming observatories similar to the stone circles in Europe. Everywhere I look I see similarities. Shamans all over the world from indigenous tribes have similar beliefs and shape-shift in dream-like states to animals. The Celtic and ancient Briton Druids had such Shamans. The Native Americans and the Saami Shaman of Lapland all worked closely with nature and animal spirits. Scholars will dismiss Atlantis as a fable designed by Plato to make a point. This may well be the case, but there is a lot of evidence for emergence of civilisation from one place, or a global civilisation. Not much is known about ancient history and Atlantis is said to have existed as far back as 9000 BC. Archaeologists will argue that lack of evidence, is evidence. A lot can be lost in 11000 years - I say, 'Keep digging!'

The Druids, Egyptians and many other civilizations are said to have gained their knowledge from a much older pre-eminent civilisation. Common folklore and as mentioned, common practices around the globe, support this thesis. If this is the case, then what happened to that civilization? The Atlantis myth sounds more and more plausible.

The Celtic Holy Grail Quest

In writing this chapter I have found my own personal Atlantis. It has always been there waiting for me, in the works of Francis Bacon, both modern and old, in Picasso's art, but most of all in the poetry of Miguel Ajeno. If you go in search of utopia you may not find what you expect. I have found a rich kingdom in Ajeno's poetry. What a mighty civilization it must once have been before time took its toll.

David Stocks

Chapter 34 Deceptive Perception and Symmetry of Illusion

Each trail on my Grail Quest brings a new thread, tying into an ever more complex Celtic knot. Closer examination of complexity however, brings simplicity. Although the knot is intricate, a lot of the weave is repeated, for often different threads end at the same juncture. My Celtic Grail quest is becoming one of symmetry, an endless knot repeating in an eternal ring. No matter where the starting point is and the twists and turns taken along the way, the same clues are revealed. To further my quest I need to analyse the repeating information I have found and solve the Celtic riddles hidden therein.

Trees have played a big part of my life since beginning this quest and play a key role in Celtic life. Looking at Celtic lore, a tree of significance is the silver birch. It is the first tree in the Ogham tree alphabet, 'Beithe.' Its slender beauty and silken silver bark gives it the title of 'The lady of the woods.' It is hardy and quick to colonise barren rocky slopes, laid bare by retreating glaciers. It is also one of the earliest to sprout new leaves in the springtime. Because of these properties it is associated with rebirth. Again there is symmetry on my quest, for being born again appears to be central to my quest. It is used for purification of gardens and to celebrate Beltane (the coming of summer, fire festival), Samhain (Halloween). The

The Celtic Holy Grail Quest

broomsticks that are famously associated with witches are traditionally made from birch. Witches flying on broomsticks are actually a legacy of the shamanic flights made by the Druids. Symmetry appears once again, for Shamans have just been discussed in the previous chapter. These flights are 'flights of the mind,' where Druids, witches, Siberian Shamans etc. would fast and then take some form of hallucinogenic drug. The mind would then be set free to go on a spiritual journey. I strongly recommend that no one either fasts or imbibes dangerous or illegal drugs. The Druids etc., who practised this, had a wealth of experience and knowledge on how to practise Shamanic flights. I have mentioned hallucinogens; this is a modern term and scientists will have you believe that they produce hallucinations. This may be? I cannot answer that. There is no doubt that the brain is affected, but there may be more to it than hallucination. They could trigger the right chemistry in the brain to allow the experienced to take Shamanic flights through the sky, or shape-shift to the form of an animal? To build more symmetry into this section, the nearest safe way to experience flights out of the body is during the hypnogogic state between sleeping and waking, a common theme that keeps recurring.

The name Birch is said to be derived from the Sanskrit word bhurga (a tree whose bark is used for writing upon). In Finland during the war it was used for just such a purpose, being both letter and envelope, having good waterproof properties. It also ties in with the idea of fate, which I will discuss in greater detail later in this book. The practice of Nadi (Sanskrit) or Naadi (Tamil) is a form of astrology going back as far as 2000 years. At this time great sages inscribed on palm leaves and possibly bark detailed descriptions of people's lives yet to come. They were able to break through into the future and read a person's life that was yet to be born. Readings are given based upon thumb prints. Accounts that I have read of such readings have been remarkably accurate. Go on recommendations if you are to have your own Nadi reading. The Tamil term Naadi means 'in search of,' which is quite apt as I am searching for the Grail. I have not had a Nadi reading, perhaps I will in the future? Such a reading would not tell me where to find the Grail, but it would tell me if I am to succeed in finding it.

One thing I have learnt so far is everything is perceived on an individual basis. What to us may seem a hallucinogenic trip - to an ancient Druid or a Native American it is a Shamanic flight. So what we perceive is real, or is it? The Grail is very elusive; to find it I may have to alter my way of thinking. Ask questions of my perception. Question the very questions I am asking. As one layer of reality unfolds, another layer is peeled back underneath it.

Below I have used a classic optical illusion to illustrate different ways of perceiving an experience. See what you make of it.

The Celtic Holy Grail Quest

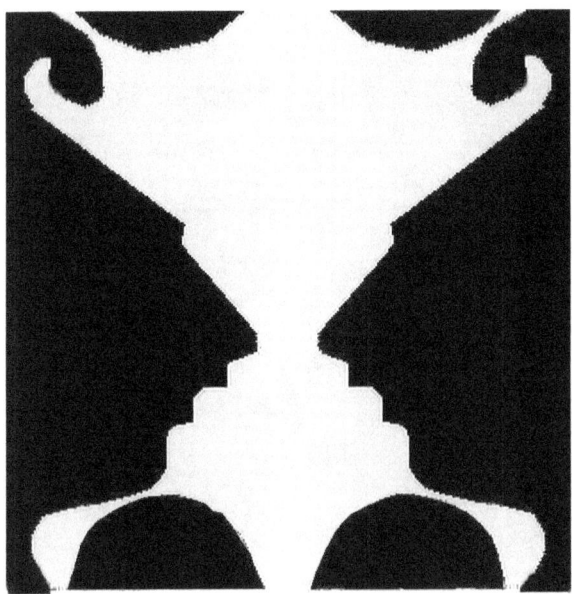

There are two possible interpretations of this image, one of a cup or a chalice, or another of the profile of two faces looking at each other.

If I fill in the detail of which these two images are actually made up, within you will find the profiles of stone carved Green Men. In the middle can be found the Holy Grail. This is quite an apt image, for it represents something at once hidden which has to be uncovered to be found. Such is the mystery of the Grail. It also represents something that is hard to grasp, for the Grail occupies the void in-between the two Green Men, almost within reach, yet impossible to touch. It is also relevant that the Grail can be seen between two figures of the Green Man.

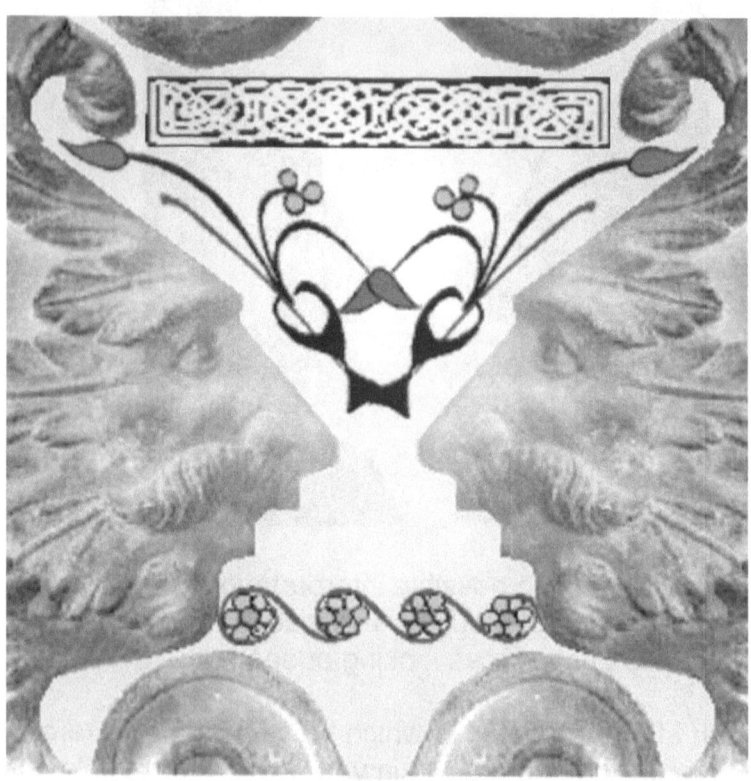

The Celtic Holy Grail Quest

Chapter 35 Languedoc and the Cathars

Continuing with the theme of coincidences that occur once you have set foot on the Grail path; I was led to a place of Grail significance. It occurred at the time of my wedding anniversary and my wife, Sue, suggested that we go to Carcassonne in Languedoc, the southernmost region of France. Carcassonne is an intact mediaeval fortress-enclosed city of towers and ramparts, the type of place Sue knew that I liked to visit. I just so happened to have started reading Christopher Dawes' excellent book entitled 'Rat Scabies and the Holy Grail,' about Rat Scabies (original drummer of the Damned) and his quest for the Holy Grail. I knew from this and numerous other sources that Rennes-le-Château lay in this region; a place steeped in mystery and a place where many Grail seekers think the Holy Grail lies hidden. I am not going to refute this and maybe a Christian version of the Grail is hidden there, but I am very sceptical about it. It is however a very interesting story of an eccentric priest, Knights Templar and Gnostic Cathars. No grail quest would be complete without visiting there and so I gladly agreed to go to Carcassonne. I didn't leave Carcassonne empty handed, however, for there were a number of enticing clues I picked up on my visit to this medieval region in the South of France.

It was the weekend starting Friday 28th April 2006 and very early in the Grail hunting season. We arrived at our destination, a little farmhouse just on the outskirts of Carcassonne. It backed onto vineyards with magnificent views of the walls and towers of the city. We spent the first day wandering through the streets of Carcassonne, transported back in time to when ladies and knights wandered the streets and minstrels played tunes, recounting tales of valour. Those tales may well have included the grail legend, as portrayed by Chrétien de Troy in his Perceval (or History of the Grail), or shortly afterwards by Robert de Boron's 'Joseph of Arimathea,' which ties the legend neatly into the Christian Celtic Church.

It was Chrétien, working in the court of Richard the Lionheart, that first brought forth images of the Round Table and Camelot. In Perceval (History of the Grail), Chrétien claimed to be only reworking material he had found in an old manuscript. Philip de Flanders commissioned Perceval, which remained uncompleted, his last work. There is no doubt that Chrétien was drawing on Celtic mythology, which led to many of the unusual marvels and mysteries of the tale. In Chrétien's tale the Grail or 'Graal' was a dish wide enough to carry a fish (could it be the Salmon of Knowledge?) It was carried in by a beautiful maiden in a procession through the Fisher King's hall and it blazed so brightly that it put out the light of the candles and stars.

In Chrétien's original working of the tale, the Grail or Graal is notably a dish, which somewhat

The Celtic Holy Grail Quest

unusually contains a consecrated wafer intended for the King's father. This suggests that Chrétien had trouble weaving the original Celtic story into Christian beliefs, as a bowl big enough for a large fish is an unusual container for a wafer. It was more than likely drawn from something of Celtic origin, perhaps one of the many cauldrons to be found in the otherworld that were imbued with magical properties?

In 1191, monks of Glastonbury disinterred the bodies of a Bronze age Chieftain and his Queen. They were identified as none other than King Arthur and Guinevere, as they bore marks of the cross on their bodies. This made Glastonbury the site of Avalon. Tradition has it that Joseph of Arimathea brought Christianity and possibly the Virgin mother herself, to Britain within a decade of Jesus' death, with the first Christian church in the world being a small circular wattle structure at Glastonbury.

Robert de Boron in Joseph of Arimathea brings the Grail legend more up to date as the chalice used by Jesus at the Last Supper and also used to catch drops of blood from the dying body of Christ on the cross. In this he makes mention of the 'Vale of Averon,' possibly the Vale of Avalon.

The church remained silent on the subject of the Grail. At around 1200, Pope innocent III began a not so innocent fourth crusade, which with the cunning intervention of the Venetians led to the sacking and pillaging of Constantinople, uniting the church as one and thus declaring Rome's supremacy as the holy centre of the church. Symmetry and coincidence again bears its head, for it was a later Pope innocent (Pope Innocent X), that Francis Bacon produced a study of, as referred to in a previous chapter.

So what has all this to do with Languedoc and the Cathars? Well, after the sacking of Constantinople, there was one irritant left to the church, the Cathars, whose Gnostic beliefs could have more holy credence than the Roman Catholic Church. The origin of the name Cathar more than likely came from a Greek word meaning 'Pure Ones.' The elders of the Cathars were called the Perfecti. The term Gnostic was derived from the Greek Gnostikos (one who has Gnosis or 'Secret Knowledge.')
The Perfecti were initiated into the deeper (secret) doctrines, of which the main mass of believers (credentes) knew nothing. The Perfecti donned simple black robes with cord belts. They surrendered all their worldly goods to the community and led dedicated lives following the doctrines of Christ and his Apostles. They devoted themselves to purity, prayer, preaching and charitable work.

The Cathars believed that within mankind existed a divine spark of creation, which was held in captivity and corrupted within the physical body and world. They believed that the world had not

The Celtic Holy Grail Quest

been created by the true God, but by a lesser god called the Demiurge, who they associated with Satan. They believed that they were trapped in this corrupt and polluted world created by the Demiurge and ruled by his minions.

Liberation from the corrupt physical realm was sought by the Cathars. They believed in reincarnation; those unable to achieve liberation during their current mortal journey were reborn to continue the struggle in the next life.

It was the failing of the Catholic church to supplant the Cathars' belief in the reincarnation of Christ, rather than the Catholic Church's belief in the resurrection of Christ, that ultimately led to Pope innocent III's crusade and wholesale massacre of the Cathars from 1209 and for many decades onwards.

Now some scholars and Grail hunters believe that the Cathars secreted away a treasure during their annihilation by the Pope's troops, one that they had brought from Jerusalem itself and which may have even been the Holy Grail.

So that is the Cathar connection of which I will go into more detail later, but what of Rennes-le-Château? Well that is an even more peculiar story and for that I needed to visit the small hilltop village in person, in the proper tradition of a Grail quester.

David Stocks

Back to our weekend break. We walked along the ramparts of the wall encircling Carcassonne town, taking in the magnificent views of the surrounding countryside and planned our trip into the Cathar region and Rennes-le-Château the next day.

We set off early on Saturday in a hired car and drove along the sometimes treacherous roads of the French Pyrenees, through a spectacular Gorge, which appeared to drop away into infinity and more often than not was only a single track. After stopping off at an authentic little auberge for a superb lunch, we made our way up a windy track to the tiny village of Rennes-le-Château.

Time to bring you up to date with the mystery surrounding Rennes-le-Château and a certain humble priest. The priest's name was Francois Berenger Sauniere and he had become a bit of a thorn in the side of the republican authorities, as he was ferverantly Royalist in his beliefs. Most people believe he was posted to Rennes-le-Château to get him out of the way. It was a ramshackle little village that Sauniere arrived in, to take up his position as Abbe Sauniere. The church was even more dilapidated, the roof unleaded and full of leaks. Sauniere's Royalist leanings led to his pay being suspended for several months and he was forced to rent a tiny room in the village when he first moved in. Eventually, after a number of months, his pay was reinstated and on that meagre salary he was able to hire a young 18 year old housekeeper, Madame Dernarnaud. With

The Celtic Holy Grail Quest

a small bequeathed sum from his predecessors, he had the two biggest holes in the church roof repaired and then a couple of years later he received a further 3000 francs from the Comtesse de Chambord, which he used for further renovation work.

Now things really started to get interesting and mightily confused. Complaining about a crack in the altar stone, Sauniere instructed his builders to extract the stone from its supporting pillars, whereupon he found some parchments concealed within one of the pillars which was hollow. Although the existence of the parchments is undoubted, the exact location of the parchments is open to debate as it appears the column was not so hollow after all. Two of the parchments were Latin passages from the Bible. Sauniere read the texts and found inconsistencies with the alignment of some of the letters. He tried to decode them all unsuccessfully and a couple of years later he showed them to his superior, the Bishop of Carcassonne. The Bishop instructed him to take the letters to Paris and was given a letter of introduction to the Director of Seminary at St Sulpice church who had expertise in ecclesiastical palaeography - in other words he might be able to decrypt the stuff.

No one knows whether Sauniere even went to Paris, or if he did, what occurred there. What everyone knows is, that soon after that time Sauniere went on a spending spree that lasted the rest of his life. He totally renovated the church of St Marie Madeline, introducing lots of gilt, stained glass windows, carvings and an assortment of the bizarre and unusual religious trappings; one notable feature being a boggle-eyed demon glaring balefully through the church doorway. Above the door he had carved the unusual words for a place of worship, 'Terribilis est locus iste' (This is a terrible place). On the basis of the great wealth amassed by Sauniere and the many exotic parties he held attended by many notable personages, it is assumed that the decrypted parchments led Sauniere to vast quantities of hidden treasure and perhaps even the fabled Holy Grail itself!

We arrived in Rennes-le-Château, a sleepy little village, outside Grail hunting season and made our way to the church of St Mary Madeline and entered under the foreboding script 'Terribilis est locus iste.' We were immediately confronted by 'boggle eyes' himself, the carved demon, guarding the inner doorway. I crouched down and stared into those demonic eyes, a staring contest I was never going to win, as those eyes were fixed in place for eternity. However with that encounter I did indeed feel that 'This place is terrible.' With a shudder I stepped into the main church beyond, darkness engulfed me and I looked towards a distant stained glass window, the only source of light. A dark cross was silhouetted against the multicoloured background, like a black bat flying out in a sunset sky.

The Celtic Holy Grail Quest

Not being a seasoned Grail hunter I didn't have the regulatory equipment pack i.e. a torch, - I immediately noticed this, because I couldn't see much of the eclectic mix of elaborately pained and sculpted decorations that adorned the church interior - spade, metal detector, lock pick, rope, sub-aqua equipment (don't ask), night vision goggles, geiger counter, dowsing rods, thermal imaging device and holy water. I didn't even have so much as a single sonic screwdriver on me. I felt unworthy, Indiana Jones I was not and I certainly didn't carry a whip. So unequipped, a virgin Rennes treasure hunter, I ventured deep into the dark interior of the church.

The coldness of the place enfolded me in its clammy grasp; I felt my body temperature drop and was engulfed with a vacuous feeling of emptiness. It wasn't so much an evil sensation but more one of despair, one with which I could associate of there being nothing there. It felt like a depressive void, a church that sucked the life out of your soul. It may not be noticed by everyone who enters that domain, but to a depressive person who is sensitised to that kind of feeling it was all too obviously present.

I didn't (couldn't) spend long in that place, unable to make out many of its features in the dim light, so I hurried out to the sanctuary that lay outside (not inside) the church.

David Stocks

Following on from the church we took the obligatory tour of the Presbytery and the Villa Bethania; I kept lagging back and examining walls and floors for secret passages and trapdoors. I would on occasion stamp my foot to see if the floor was hollow and feel along cracks in the walls for possible secret doors. This irrational behaviour would promote chance encounters with other tourists, suspiciously examining the rooms in a very similar manner to myself. We would look each other up and down and try to appear nonchalant about our activities; the stamping would be just to get warmth into our feet for example. There was no such thing as a normal tourist at Rennes-le-Château, all were infected with Grail fever, and you could see it by the feverish look in their eyes.

Having found no secret hideaways in the Villa, we went out into the gardens surrounded by a wall, the top of which gave stunning views of the valleys below. The site of Rennes-le-Château was on a very prominent hilltop, just the sort of place for buried treasure. The wall ended in the Tour Magdala, an impressive square tower that made up the final promontory of Rennes-le-Château hilltop. Inside the tower was an empty tiled room, of which I took pictures. I hoped later to find some kind of significant geometric pattern hidden in the layout of the tiles. Later studies of these photographs failed to reveal any code laid out in them and certainly no pointing arrows saying 'This way to the Grail,' but a true Grail seeker must

The Celtic Holy Grail Quest

explore all avenues.

We climbed the spiral staircase to the top of the tower, a vantage point from which all the domain below appeared subservient to those in command on the Tour Magdala. Could it be from here where Sauniere mapped out the true resting place of the Grail? From here, can the unseen be seen?

Despite a lengthy period of time at Rennes-le-Château (a day denotes an exhaustive amount of Grail hunting time to me), I found no trace of the Holy Grail, or any clues as to its location. People have spent years searching for treasure at Rennes-le-Château; the place is supposedly riddled with tunnels. If those determined Grail hunters were unable to find so much as a gold coin in all their explorations, then I was not going to waste any more time physically searching that location.

So what of the mysteries surrounding the parchments? These parchments have since been decoded, the first being a fairly simple code made out of upraised letters that decodes as:

'A Dagobert II Roi et a Sion est ce tresor et ill est la mort.'
('This treasure belongs to King Dagobert II and to Sion and he is there dead.')

Great! If it killed King Dagobert, who was a mighty Morovian king blessed with supernatural powers, then I, a mere mortal, had better tread carefully. He was murdered by his own men three years after acceding to the Austrasian crown.

As for Sion, it was a mystical order formed on mount Sion in the holy land at the time of the last Crusade.

The second parchment was a lot more difficult to decode and involved passing it through a devious encryption table called the Vigenere Table (twice) and a complex game of chess with one knight and two chessboards. This was more like a code and decrypted it read:

'Bergere pas de tentation. Que Poussin Teniers gardent le clef. Pas DCLXXXI. Par la croix et ce cheval de Dieu j'achevece daemon de gardien a midi. Pommes bleues.'

(Sheperdesss no temptation. That Poussin [and] Teniers holds the key. Peace 681. By the cross and this horse of God I destroy this Demon Guardian at midday. Blue apples.')

The Tenniers painting could be one of several versions he did of the Temptation of Anthony, but the Poussin painting seemed to relate to a painting 'The Shepherds of Arcadia.' This shows a pastoral scene in which four figures, one of which is a shepherdess, are gathered around an ancient tomb inscribed with the words 'Et In Arcadia Ego.' The scene was originally thought to be an artistic

The Celtic Holy Grail Quest

image and not based on a real location. In the 1970s however a lonely roadside tomb was shown to match the image and surroundings in the painting. The tomb has since been destroyed, but old photographs show the tomb with the unmistakable contour of the Rennes-le-Château mountain as one of the mountains in the background. This place can still be visited and is on many a Holy Grail quester's itinerary.

The 'Blue Apples' is thought to be associated with a mystical effect of light that occurs once a year in the St Marie Madeline church in Rennes-le-Château. On 17th January each year in the low winter sun, shimmering apple shaped blue dots of light hover in the air within the confines of the Church. Rather spookily 17th January is the date on which both Berenger Sauniere and Marie Blanchefort died. This Rennes-le-Château mystery seems to involve a lot of dead people. Does the Grail only come to those who are prepared to die?

A lot of speculation has surrounded the two parchments, the codes they have revealed and the treasure that Sauniere is supposed to have found. Much of it, very in-depth, but of greatest interest to me, is the Cathars and in particular the siege of Monsegur. The night before the Cathar castle of Monsegur fell to the holy crusade, a small band of four Cathars (or possibly even Knights Templar) are supposed to have smuggled out a very secret and holy treasure, one that is rumoured to have been brought back from the

David Stocks

Holy land.

Now the Knights Templar keep appearing on this Holy Grail Quest and have long been rumoured to be Guardians of the Grail. Many people have searched for the roots of the Knights Templar and believe they were founded on the much older Order of Sion. Links have also been made to Ancient Egyptian civilizations, Myan, Aztec and Druidic traditions. Wherever I look all these legends merge into one and support the thesis for a common origin for ancient doctrines and religion. Some chapters of the Masons are said to have Templar roots, with modern day Templars bringing the wisdom full circle and being founded on those very Masonic beliefs. Again there is symmetry.

Whatever was hidden at Montsegur is no longer there, but my feeling is that this treasure is the very same treasure that lies at the heart of the Rennes-le-Château mystery, for Montsegur lies within a few miles of Rennes-le-Château.

There is much, much more legend and myth associated with Rennes-le-Château, but looking at the words inscribed over the church entrance, 'Terribilis est locus iste' ('This place is terrible') and the deaths of both Sauniere and Blanchefort on 17th January, I feel there is a very dark side to the treasure that is to be found.

For the rest of our weekend break in Languedoc we travelled deep into the heart of the region and

The Celtic Holy Grail Quest

visited many spectacular ruins of Cathar castles. From these explorations into this mystical landscape I can well believe there is a secret to be found, but not one I wish to pursue myself. Oh wanderers on this devious labyrinth of the Grail, leave me here if you desire this dark token that portrays itself as the Holy Grail and seek it in the hidden lands of the Cathars. Continue with me those who seek the true Grail, for this journey is far from complete, but this is an important step along the way.

To learn something of the nature of the Grail from this trip is to understand the common origins of the Legend, at once Christian, Gnostic, Egyptian, Celtic, and Aztec. I believe this treasure has been concealed within layers of ancient wisdom. Perhaps the Gnostic belief that the divine power is within and must be found by searching the self, is a key clue to further me on this quest?

Chapter 36 Strange goings on in the Peak District

The Peak District may not have the seething intrigue of the Cathars, but it has a much more ancient and powerful history, full of primeval forces. Sue and I visited it on a number of occasions; on one such occasion we stayed in a little village called Elton with some long time friends of ours, Jane and Tim. Sue has known Jane all her life; she is tall, slim and dark haired, a very down to earth, go-with-the-flow sort of person. Tim, Jane's partner, runs a riding stable and also rears sheep. He is of average height, sturdily built with short brown hair and the sort of face that is always on the verge of breaking in to a smile. A nicer couple you could not hope to meet.

We stayed in a little bed and breakfast located on the main street running through Elton. Sue and I had the luxury of an old four poster bed, which Jane and Tim had insisted on us having. The mattress was so high on the bed that a set of steps led up to it. It was a grand experience going to bed later and we felt like a King and Queen striding up to our bed, seemingly in the clouds. We could only hope that things did not go bump in the night, as it was a long way down.

Before blissful sleep embraced us in our heavenly bed, we strode out of the village in the early evening and made our way across the fields

The Celtic Holy Grail Quest

toward Birchover and its pub, the Druid Inn. The tangled skein casts its web over the Grail quest again, for Birchover derives its name from 'the ridge where birch trees grow.' As explored in previous chapters, the Birch has Great significance to the Celts, one of which is rebirth. Rebirth plays an ever more significant part on my quest for the Grail. The Druid Inn naturally has Druid connotations, largely derived from the Rowter Rocks situated above the Inn. These huge grit stone rocks were said to rock from side to side before the collection of silt and earth over the ages. Passages and a tightly hewn out cave, was where the ancient Druids were said to have held their ceremonies. Such chambers were again associated with rebirth, with initiates shutting themselves off from the outside world and emerging with an understanding of reality. Having been confined to such a tomb, they would also have lost their fear of death and were reborn. Our evening walk led us to Birchover across the top of a hill, - on which lay an ancient stone circle - over dry stone walls, and down into the valley below. A final scramble took us up the steep incline on the other side of the valley and deposited us at our destination, a little back lane into Birchover and the Druid Inn.

A log fire was blazing in the hearth and we sat enjoying delicious home made food cooked to traditional recipes, while supping pints chosen from the excellent range of real ales. I considered the life of an initiate not bad, but I did forgo my chance of a night's sleep in the Druid chamber in favour of the prospect of the four poster bed. We had a long restful evening inventing ghost stories, regaling each other with accounts of spooky happenings at the stone circle we had passed on route to the Druid. The cold stone chamber was going to prove much more inviting than the journey back.

All this talk had its inevitable effect, when full of food and drink we tottered out of the Druid to make our return journey in the dark. A sinister cloak cast itself upon the dark hills and hidden depths of the surrounding Peak District countryside. Conjurations of the mind manifest themselves in the darkness of time, places as old as the land itself lay hidden within its folds. The rationale of the group kept the demons at bay, but more tricks were played on the mind as we stumbled on hidden stones and snagged ourselves on outstretched branches. When once there was safety in numbers, group hysteria led to dysfunction and hallucination. All manner of the mind's beasts now lay in wait for us.

The further away from the Druid we went, the darker it became, the only light being the stars above us that shone out with a brilliance we were not used to seeing from our urban homes. The journey became interminable, whispers of wind at our ears chased us all the way. More by luck than chance, we stumbled upon the stone circle. It was a hallowed place, a place that had not been

The Celtic Holy Grail Quest

frequented at night since the time of the Druids. We stood in awe, like startled rabbits caught in the beam of headlights. We had strayed off the path of time and stumbled back through millennia. Carefully we walked around the stones, looking to the heavens as we did so. Gossamer threads of starlight shimmered upon a celestial stone spinning wheel and galaxies spun around its axis. We were in the presence of great power bridging time and space. We had stumbled upon the secret workings of the universe but were prey to ourselves. The fear once again clenched our hearts and our fight or flight mechanism kicked in. Leaving the inner workings of the universe behind us, we made haste across olden hills and back to the safety of our Bed and Breakfast.

I spent a restless night sleeping in the old four poster bed, adrift in time, carried through space on an ancient craft. It was a sturdy bed carved out of oak, a wood sacred to the Druids, and I lay there all alone in a sea of stars. I knew that we were not alone in the universe, however, as I could feel the presence of others and for that night only I could almost touch them.

Breakfast was served down in the cafe below; of a similar nature to the one I had visited at Market Rasen on my first motorbike. I was transported back to a 50s cafe once again! The walls were adorned with metal plates advertising all sorts of products from a bygone era. Even the till was an ornate silver mechanical one, displaying prices in

David Stocks

old money. Again I was trapped in a time bubble and we were served the most magnificent full English breakfast seated by the side of an old wood fire.

That trip was magical, one I will always treasure. More research on the stone circle we encountered revealed that it contained the tallest standing stones in the Peak District, with the tallest standing stone being 2.1 metres in height. Before the stones were re-erected and cast in concrete in 1936, the tallest stone measured 3.5 metres long. The stone circle is known as the 'Nine Stones Close,' although only four remain standing. An alternate name for them is the 'Grey Ladies,' who are rumoured to dance at midnight. It would have been about that time when we returned from the Druid Inn and perhaps we witnessed their dance, spinning the stars on their wheel and dancing the dance of the spheres? Alternative folklore says that by moonlight the stones spin and dance.

I have returned to the area many times since. On one occasion Sue, my parents and I visited another stone circle, the Nine Ladies (to be distinguished from the Grey Ladies) early one spring morning. This is located on Stanton Moor, not far from Birchover, with the stones being very small in comparison to the Grey Ladies. Sue and my mother performed a spontaneous sun worship dance, welcoming the day's sun as it cast its rays over the stones, leaving long fingers of shadows behind. A long hot summer was to follow and

The Celtic Holy Grail Quest

thankfully Sue and my mother were not cast in stone; legend has it that a fiddler and nine ladies came to dance on the moor one Sunday morning, a sacrilegious act that had them turned to stone.

The Grey Ladies stone circle lies but a step or stride away from Robin Hood's stride. Legend has it that Robin Hood strode the distance between the towering stones that made up Robin Hood's stride. This was a monumental feat as the stones are 15 metres apart, but maybe not such a feat for Cerrunous (the Green Man), from which the Robin Hood legend was possibly derived. Birchover has played host to filming, notably the film 'The Princess Bride.' This is a tongue-in-cheek fairytale and has been compared to 'Monty Python and the Holy Grail' in terms of its humour. Robin Hood's stride is one of the locations used in the film; perhaps the Grail is having a laugh at my attempts to obtain it or just maybe by participating in the joke I will find that elusive Grail? Each step on this journey is full of surprises and the Grail turns up where you least expect it.

There is a power in Britain's old stones, one that is no longer understood, one that may someday bring man back into harmony with nature in the Celtic way of life.

An interesting find on Stanton Moor in 1889 was that of a tiny 2 inch high cup. They have been previously known as incense cups and found alongside those of funerary urns. An incense cup is an inaccurate description however. The contents have been found to contain small fragments of burnt bone, but these could easily have been picked up elsewhere in a burial site. Little is known about these cups and it is thought they may be symbolic containers for carrying food into the afterlife. Similar Pigmy cups have been found at Nith Lodge Cairn in Scotland. Along with triangular scored patterns encircling the top and bottom sections of the outside, they bear a five pointed star on the base.

Nith Lodge Cairn is circa 2000 - 1600 BC and is typical of early Bronze Age. Five pointed stars have become known as pentagrams, with the earliest reference being from the Sumerians as pictograms for the word UB (corner, angle, nook; a small room, cavity, hole; pitfall). Sumerian being the earliest recorded language from about 3000 BC, the pentagram has been a symbol of significance throughout the ages. It has more recently been associated with devil worship, but early Christians used it as a symbolic device, representing the five wounds of Christ.

So what of its association with the Grail? The Knights Templar used the Pentagram symbol in connection with the temple of Solomon in Jerusalem. It was used as the seal of the city of Jerusalem and known as the 'Seal of Solomon' as far back as the 4th Century BC. The symbol represented infinity, connectedness and oneness. These are all recurring themes throughout the

The Celtic Holy Grail Quest

book. In the 14th century poem, 'Sir Gawain and the Green Knight,' Sir Gawain (one of Arthur's most noble knights), bears the pentagram as his coat of arms. In the extracted verse below, it shows significant ties to the temple of Solomon and the endless knot.

And I intend to tell you, though I tarry therefore, why the Pentangle is proper to this prince of knights.
It is a symbol which Solomon conceived once
To betoken holy truth, by its intrinsic right,
For it is a figure which has five points,
And each line overlaps and is locked with another;
And it is endless everywhere, and the English call it,
In all the land, I hear, the Endless Knot.

The endless knot is seen in another form as the Celtic knot, endlessly interweaving and repeating itself into infinity. The pentagram was important to the Celts as a symbol of the underworld and that of the Goddess Morrigan. Because the pentagram is a five pointed star and created by drawing five lines without the pen leaving the paper, it has great significance with the powerful number 5. In case you were wondering about the arrival of another significant number other than 23, 2 + 3 = 5. There it is again. Below are some associations with the number 5:-

Body: We commonly note five senses - sight, hearing, smell, touch and taste.

David Stocks

We have five toes on each of our feet and five fingers on each of our hands.
Religion: In Christianity, five were the wounds of Christ on the cross.
There are five pillars of the Muslim faith and five daily times of prayer.
Medieval virtues: Five were the virtues of the medieval knight - generosity, courtesy, chastity, chivalry and piety as symbolised in the pentagram device of Sir Gawain.
Witchcraft: The Wiccan Kiss is fivefold - feet, knees, womb, breasts, lips - blessed be.
The quintessential spirit is represented by the five triangles on the outside of the pentagram and it is these five triangles that can be seen on the bottom of the pigmy cup.
To the Gnostics it was a blazing star; along with the crescent moon it symbolised the night sky and magic. To the Egyptians in Egypt, it was a symbol of the 'underground womb;' it bore a symbolic relationship to the concept of the pyramid form.

Again all the strands that have been woven are tying into the same knot, this time the endless knot of the Pentagram. Researching the endless Celtic knot and that of Morrigan, I am now drawn to the power of three. For Morrigan is an Irish triple goddess:

Ana, the fertility maiden; Badb, the boiling mother cauldron, producer of life; and Macha, the death-crone symbolized by the carrion-devouring raven. Morrigan is the mistress of the Cauldron, 'The

The Celtic Holy Grail Quest

Cauldron of Rebirth.' Being reborn is of continuing significance to my quest. So is that of the endless knot, the continuous cycle, infinity. Another aspect of Morrigan is that of a raven. Raven bones have been found within burial sites and are significant to death. With death takes flight the raven, foreteller of doom and like the banshee, harbinger of death. Then through the cauldron the spirit is reborn.

I return to Gawain and his importance to the Grail quest. In medieval tales, he was a knight of the most chivalrous kind. In terms of the Grail, he was in pursuit of the Grail, whose tail remained unfinished in Chrétien De Troy's original 'Perceval' (le Conte du Graal). He is often associated with Cuchulainn, who like Gawain wore a magical belt rendering him invincible. In Malory's 'Morte d' Arthur,' Sir Gawain encounters the female enchantress, Morgan le Fay, the half sister of King Arthur. Strikingly there are similarities between Morgan and Morrigan. Usually Morgan appeared as a beautiful young woman, sometimes as an old hag, notably in Gawain and the Green Knight. Morrigan also had the same ability to shape-shift between young and old, beautiful and ugly. Like Morrigan, she was able to transform herself to look like any animal or inanimate object. One more interesting clue concerning Gawain - he was known as a great healer - is shown in this extract from Perceval below:

> **Of wounds and healing lore**
> **Did Sir Gawain know more**
> **Than any man alive?**

David Stocks

To make the sick knight thrive,
A herb to cure all pain
That in a hedge had lain
He spied, and thence he plucked it.

There is a painting of Gawain meeting a wounded knight at King Ludwig's Bavarian fairytale castle of Neuschwanstein. On my last trip there it was hidden in mist, until I rose above the clouds to see heavenly turrets and parapets hovering in the air. What more fitting place for a Grail castle could there be? Perhaps the Grail can be found in some secret chamber there? I don't know. But by following Gawain's story and that of the Fisher King, a property of the Grail might well be healing. It is towards this aim I continue my quest, for to heal people's spirits is what I seek and I look to the Grail for guidance in this. I now understand that I must heal my own wounds inflicted on my mind, before I can help others.

I wonder about the journey through Grail legends that a small burial vessel took me on. A mere two inches in diameter, yet could such a vessel hold the key to the Grail? A tiny cup is a cup, is it not?

The Celtic Holy Grail Quest

Chapter 37 Dream Siren

Summer dreams wandered the empty hallways of my mind. These dreams were so real I had trouble distinguishing reality from fiction on waking. On one instance I had a dream visitation. It was the image of someone calling out to me from the past. All I could see was a face shrouded in mist, a face I hadn't seen since I last worked as a computer consultant. A gentle smile beckoned me back through the folds of time, back to where this journey began. She came to me as an angel in my dreams.

I awoke from this dream with her image clear in my head. Her name was Jules and she was a colleague of mine when I last worked in computing. We worked closely together and all day I could not get Jules out of my head. My past was calling me.

I had the same dream the next night. On waking I realised I had to accept the existence of my past and get back in touch with Jules. It was an awakening of an old spirit that I had shut away in a closet for many years.

Plucking up my courage I rang Jules, but was disappointed when I only got through to an answering machine. Nervously I left a message on the machine and truly never expected to hear any more from her.

David Stocks

It came as a shock to me when I got a call from Jules that evening and heard her vibrant voice on the other end of the line. We chatted for quite a while and caught up on each other's history for the last five years. At the end of the conversation we agreed to meet up again.

We met in a car park close to where Jules now lived. I had to take a second look, for when Jules stepped out of her car, it was a totally different Jules to the one I remembered. She now had long braided hair down to her waist (she had shoulder length dark hair the last time I saw her) and walked with a confidence I had not seen in her before. We went back to her house, where we resumed on catching up on old times.

I told her about my decline into depression and psychosis, following my mental breakdown. I told her it had been induced by the stress of the computing job and the long hours away from home. I then recounted my experiences in different jobs I had undertaken since then. Jules herself had moved on and was now a senior web programmer/developer in a large corporation. She had been at this job for a number of years now and had made a lot of new friends, living life to the full.

We talked for hours and our friendship was renewed, as if the five years apart had never happened. I eventually had to leave, but we made

The Celtic Holy Grail Quest

plans to see each other again the following week.

Over a period of time our friendship blossomed, until it reached a point where we became more then friends. This put me in a difficult situation for my wife had never been anything but loyal to me and had looked after me selflessly during my years of depression. But my feelings for Jules had grown too strong and after much fretting I left my home and refuge for the last twelve years. I moved to a flat in another village in the Nottingham area, with a view to developing my relationship with Jules.

Together we made trips to places as a couple and I remember on one such outing, we visited Stratford to see The Tempest, Jules' favourite Shakespeare play. The performance was spectacular, but our lasting memories of it was of the part of Ariel, a sprite of magical powers, ensnared by a sorcerer to do his service. Ariel was acted so well, he could well have been a magical being from another realm. He stole the stage and posed majestically while singing in an ethereal warbling voice, that stirred the innermost emotions. A beauty to both eyes and ears, transporting us directly into Shakespeare's mystical play and ensnaring us there forever. I still cannot get that performance out of my head and it was the shared experience of that performance that brought my angel to me. She called to me from a dream and in a dream came to me.

Chapter 38 Breaking out of a mental fog

As my relationship grew stronger with Jules she encouraged me to stop taking my medication, as she thought it was dulling my senses. After careful consideration I took the bold step of coming off my medication all in one go (this is *not* recommended as a person can suffer serious side effects by doing this and may also lose any benefits - known or unknown - that the medication may be giving!)

It took a few weeks for the medication to clear out of my system and several weeks more before it was completely washed out of my body. The effect though was amazing; from taking fairly high doses of five different medications to running on none, I suddenly emerged from a mental haze. Everything around me took on a dramatic new clarity, my mind could function again. I was born again, my brain was rejuvenated, neurons were firing like a finely tuned engine. I didn't realise the severe effect the drugs were having on me until I stopped taking them. I went from being a zombie, to a fully functioning human being again.

The difficulties I had encountered while working as an assistant librarian, evaporated. Tasks I had previously found to be difficult I was now finding easy and what had been a challenging job now became almost mundane.

My mental euphoria was rudely interrupted

The Celtic Holy Grail Quest

however by a nasty virus that sent me reeling into sickness again. This virus had probably caught my body in a weak state, having come off the medication all in one go. I was attacked by headaches, weakness and stomach complaints, which resulted in me being off work again for a period of time.

It took me a while to fully recover from this virus and hence my work at the library suffered on return to work, but only for a short period. While I was on medication I had been put on extended probation as a result of my poor performance. Apart from the dip in my performance again, when I had the virus, my work had gone from poor to top notch. This unfortunately was not recognised by the management. Staff shortages had resulted in my work not being properly monitored since stopping the medication and I was not given credit for the quality or quantity of my work.

A review of my work was taken with management and a member of the County Council personnel. In this meeting it was raised that I was still being monitored, a fact I was not aware of at the time and that this would have to continue for the foreseeable future. They didn't then think my work was up to standard. This I strongly disagreed with and despite raising an objection to further monitoring and the detrimental effect that it would have on my mental health - raised through the correct procedures both to my line management and the council - I was still put on further appraisal. The result of this treatment sent me over the edge and into another mental breakdown, with a total lack of self confidence. It is difficult to explain how lack of belief can shatter the fragile confidence of a depressed person. I was a victim of circumstance; there was not enough staff to realise my fully functioning value resulting in my prior work history being taken as the standard at which I was assumed to be. The net result was long term sickness from the library, a situation I had tried to avoid. Their lack of belief fuelled doubts within me.

I was still working at the coffee shop during this period and I struggled on there for a short while with the full support of the management, who helped me a great deal. I ultimately had to give this up though, as I needed support from Jules and I decided to move in with her. This moved me away from Costa and I realised I would not be able to fit in with their working hours.
Having been living with Jules for a while I felt more mentally alert but still had lost all my confidence, preventing me from returning to the library work. With my enlightened mental state I was able to progress with the writing of this book and also explore the surrounding area more, Jules' house being located in a village called Stonnall, just outside Lichfield. These wanderings, along with trips to the Lake District, have set rise to the next few chapters and the conclusion of this story.

While the clarity of my mind had blossomed, my

The Celtic Holy Grail Quest

moods had suffered as a result of being off medication and the mood stabilisers. My mood was like a roller coaster, up one minute then down the next. It was more downs than ups however and I likened it more to the big dipper.

I took to walks around the surrounding area, often with Jules at night by the light of the stars and the moon. These walks refreshed me both mentally and physically and I was able to get more in harmony with nature, more in tune with the Celtic way of life, but I had to do something about these mood dips which were getting more severe.

Stonnall derives its name from the Saxon 'stan halh' meaning 'stony ground' and was listed as:
Stanahala, in 1143
Stanahala, in 1167
Stonhal, during the third Henry's reign.
Had my quest hit 'stony ground?'

I think not. Looking further into the history of Stonnall, the Chester road used to run through it and connect up to the old Roman road, Watling Street. The juncture of this road at High Cross with the Fosse has had earlier significance on this quest. Again I travel into the past along that old Roman road. What significance could it have? Time was yet to reveal more secrets encountered in this small Staffordshire village.
On one of my walks I picked up a stone, of which there were plenty, and cast it into the nearby Footherly Brook. In one of the Grail legends, the

David Stocks

Grail is actually a stone and with a stone I cast out my thoughts on the Grail. The ripples spread in that once still water; into the future I followed them, from my castle now in Stonnall, for an Englishman's home is his castle. From there I would sally forth, further on my Grail quest.

The Celtic Holy Grail Quest

Chapter 39 Lost in the mists of time

From a mental fog to a September fog, high up in the Lake District mountains. Jules and I found ourselves adrift in the fog shrouded peaks, on a trip we made to the Lake District, a break away from our regular lives.

The fog descended on us as we made the steep ascent up Kirkstone Pass. What was initially just thin wisps of mist became dense rolling fog, enveloping us in its clammy grasp and concealing all that lay before us. The headlights of our car barely picked out the road ahead and the vertiginous drops that awaited us around each bend. Steeper and steeper we climbed, into the unknown we ventured. We heard the engine of our Alpha Romeo Spider going from the purr of a panther to the roar of a lion as we made our ascent. This stretch of the pass was aptly named 'the struggle.'

Just as we were thinking of turning back a light shimmered in the distance, a beacon in the fog that beckoned us towards it, a ray of hope on this dark misty night. The light cast its beam through the fog, becoming ever brighter as we neared its location. Upon rounding a final bend we came to the source of the illumination. It was an old inn, a whitewashed building seeming as old as the pass itself. The Kirkstone Inn awaited us weary travellers of the night.

David Stocks

The Kirkstone Inn was located right at the top of the pass and no such remote an inn could there possibly be in all of England, and what a welcome sight it was! Parking the car we ventured out into the fog on foot across the car park through freezing blankets of mist, washing up on the shores of the inn. Opening the old latched door to the pub we were suddenly hit with a wave of heat and light. The interior of the inn was warm and cosy with an open log fire blazing in a stone hearth. An old sheepdog looked up at us as we entered, comfortable in its place by the fire. The ceiling was low and beamed, a bar stood in the corner of the room and we were greeted with a friendly smile by the barmaid as we approached.

To our delight we found that they served a piping hot mulled wine and we were soon warm and snug next to the fire, sipping our mulled wine, a warm glow flushing our cheeks. We were pleasantly surprised to find the pub frequented by other travellers on this cold night and found ourselves chatting to two friendly American men sat on the bench opposite us.

Having recognised their North American accents we enquired as to whereabouts in the states they were from.
'From Arizona,' they replied.
They were both well built, one with long wavy blonde hair who resembled a surf dude and the other had short dark hair and quite thickset features.

The Celtic Holy Grail Quest

We chatted for a while and the conversation turned to music, at which point the blonde haired guy said he played in a band.
Jules asked, 'Are you famous?'
'Only to my wife and kids,' he replied.

They left shortly afterwards, bidding us a friendly farewell as we enjoyed our second glass of mulled wine.
The friendly people and the mulled wine served to lift our spirits and, feeling warm and refreshed, we reluctantly left the inn to make our journey back.

On opening the door to leave the pub, a wave of mist swirled in through the entrance and on stepping out we were soon engulfed by the fog. Leaving the welcoming lights of the inn behind us, we ventured out into the murkiness and its cold clammy grasp.

Not a sound could be heard and the only thing visible was the lights of the inn, hazy in the depths of the fog. As we walked further away even these disappeared. Time stopped as we were cast adrift on a sea of fog, disorientated we lost all sense of direction.

We felt time slip away, all was deathly still, and only the sound of our own breathing could be heard. We stopped walking, wary of going over the edge of the steep pass.
This fog was a real pea soup'er (as we call it from where I come from) and a pretty vicious pea soup

at that. It was one that you could stand your spoon up in, one that Mum used to make that would set into green cement the next day. Our imaginations conjured up ghostly images in the fog and we were keen to break free of its clammy clasp.
We eventually found our way to the car by repeatedly pressing the key fob and homing in on the bleeps and faint traces of light emitting from it. It was more like swimming than walking, through the mist to the car.

The journey back was treacherous with the car headlights barely picking out the road ahead of us, zigzagging round hairpin bends for what seemed like an eternity until we reached the sanctuary of Ambleside.

The next day dawned clear and bright. Stepping out into the fresh morning air, we felt invigorated and decided to return to the Kirkstone Inn, to see it in the daylight.

The views were stupendous, as we made our way back up the pass, with each bend providing us with a new awe inspiring vista. The inn stood bright in the morning light and we parked our car in the car park across the way. It still being too early to partake of the inn's refreshments we decided to venture out on foot and inspect the stone from which the pass got its name. Having read about the pass, we had discovered that there was a stone up on a mountain across from the inn that had a point resembling a church's roof. In

The Celtic Holy Grail Quest

Scottish this is called 'Kirk', hence the name of the stone and the pass.

The stone stood like a lone sentry on the hillside, reminding me of the shape of a quartz crystal leaning out at a slight angle from the hillside, with its straight sides slanting to a point at the top. I marvelled at the loneliness of the rock and wandered at the geological process that must have created it. There was pride in its bearing, a rock that must have been revered through the ages. I was reminded of my Celtic quest and felt humbled by the stone, as must the Celts have been prior to the Romans who passed this way a Millennia ago. I considered this to be a sacred stone to the Celts, who admired such landmarks and venerated them in their time.

It was midday by the time we got back to the inn and started talking about the eerie fog the night before. We were then told many tales of haunting, including that of a 17th Century coachman. As with many old inns, it had no shortage of ghostly happenings. I quietly wondered if any echoes of Celtic people still wandered this lonely pass?

Chapter 40 Two guests arrive, of the feline kind

On our return from the Lake District we were plunged into a whole new role, for we were to have lodgers at Jules' house and the lodgers were cats.

Now I have lived with cats for many years in my previous home, but for Jules, cats were a whole new experience, and what an experience it was!

Before I embark on the story of the cats and our relationship with them, I will start by explaining Jules' empathy with the animal kingdom and that of fish. On moving into her house, Jules inherited a pond full of fish, Koi Carp to be precise. All through the summer months, Jules had built up a relationship with the fish, to the point that she had names for many of them, Kevin an unusually large carp, being one of them. She was able to go to the side of the pond and had the fish surfacing in front of her and kissing her hand. At feeding time they were literally eating out of her hand. Jules had an affinity with the fish and would spend many happy hours talking to them by the side of the pond. The Salmon of Knowledge however, was nowhere to be seen.

Jules has a gentle way with animals of all kinds, but she had never had cats before. Having spent many pleasant years with cats, I told her she had

The Celtic Holy Grail Quest

been missing out and that soon she would learn the delights of the feline kingdom.

The cats were to lodge with us for a few months, as a friend of ours was in-between houses and had no permanent place for them to stay. On the day of their arrival, Jules was tense. This tension did not last long however, for the cats, Tilly and Taffy, came into the house and immediately settled on two chairs in the conservatory. As you can probably tell by their names, they come from one of the Celtic heartlands, Wales.

Taffy is a ginger tom and the best way to describe him is that he resembles Garfield. Taffy I have to say has turned out to be the most affectionate cat I have ever come across. Jules picked him up and he immediately snuggled onto her shoulder and started purring like mad.

Tilly is one of the prettiest cats that I have ever seen. She is small boned and has defined cheek bones and a cute little smile, a smile that she puts to best effect with a tilt of her head (that little lost cat look), a look that we got to know better as time went by. Her fur is a delicate pattern of pale silvery grey and white.

Now you may wonder where this chapter is leading, but for those suffering from depression, cats are very therapeutic. They make great companions. For the purposes of the Grail quest, it is very important to understand the strong bonds with animals that the Celts had.

The cats settled in fairly quickly and after initial nerves they started to make it their home. If you have ever lived with cats, you will understand that it is *their* home and it is on this understanding that they let you live with them. Taffy by this time had taken to eating regularly, not only having meals, but requesting Taff snacks in-between meals. Tilly however was not getting a look in at meal times and would therefore go for long periods without a meal. This issue we addressed by leaving Tilly's food on the counter, which was out of bounds for a now hefty Taffy.

Having resolved the food issues, we addressed the sleeping arrangements. Taffy took to sleeping on our bed with us and Tilly under advice from her owner, slept on top of the bedroom wardrobe in a basket. All perfectly normal I'm sure.

As the weeks went by, Taffy began to noticeably put on weight. It was when he started to struggle to get through the cat flap, we realised that something urgent needed doing. To us, it had been good that he had been eating a lot, as it meant that he was content. We of course for health reasons, realised that he needed to go on a diet.

Now putting Taffy on a diet was not an easy thing, because Taffcat as we now called him can be very demanding as far as food is concerned. For Taffy,

The Celtic Holy Grail Quest

life revolves around his tummy, which according to him is empty most of the time. To put this into perspective I will outline a typical Taffy day.

4.00 am: Taffy stirs and makes his first pleas for breakfast. If we make the mistake of getting up to go to the toilet, Taffy is up like a shot to block us off at the stairs.

6.00 am: This is at the moment our normal getting up time for going to work. When the alarm goes off, Taffy is on his starting blocks and the minute we vacate the bed Taffy is waiting at the top of the stairs.

6.30 am: Having washed and got ready, a procedure which has Taffy following you into every room, it is downstairs and finally breakfast time. Taffy has by this time run down the stairs and is waiting in the kitchen.

Now Taffy has a slight identity crisis; instead of meowing around your feet, he starts quacking like a duck. His quacks get ever more demanding and insistent until he gets his food. I think he may have been crossed with a duck at birth.

7.00 am: Taffy having had his breakfast is now stationed in the kitchen awaiting the next person to arrive downstairs. He then starts to tell said person that he has not yet been fed and where is his breakfast? All in quacks of course.

David Stocks

10.00 am: Taffy now has not eaten for a considerable amount of time and is demanding that I, as I have been working from home, give him his mid morning snack.

12.00 midday: Taffy has lunch with me, we usually share some ham.

3.00 pm: Time for Taffy's afternoon snack. This is essential as he could pass away at any time.

6.00 pm: Time for his tea, he quacks repeatedly until he gets given a pouch of food, which he chooses himself.

6.30 pm: Time for his tea (again), as he obviously hasn't been fed yet and he tells whichever one of us who didn't feed him that he hasn't had his tea yet.

7.30 pm: Taffy quacks for more food, just on the off chance he may get some.

9.30 pm: Taffcat is on his last legs now and if he doesn't get some supper soon, he may just collapse. This he usually does, just for show.

As you can see, Taffy's world is a world of food, more food and any extra treats he may be able to scrounge in-between.

Despite vehement protestations at ever more frequent intervals, we put Taffy on a diet. Over a

The Celtic Holy Grail Quest

period of a couple of months he slimmed down to a healthy weight, but is still demanding extra food all the time.

The next episode involves Tilly's meals. Now if you remember, Tilly has her food on the counter, which was inaccessible to Taffcat. However the new slim-line Taffcat soon realised that with his new trim physique, he could now make it up to the counter. It wasn't for a while until we found Taffcat out and in the meantime Tilly had been missing out on meals.

Tilly who used to hunt for her food before she had her own supply, had now taken to catching her food again. In one great feat of hunting, which is now legendary in the feline world, she caught a magpie. This we found one morning when we came down to magpie feathers all over the lounge. You must realise Tilly is only a tiny cat and a magpie is easily as big as her.

Drastic action had to be taken; we had to move Tilly's food to a location that the new slim-line Taffcat could not reach. There was only one place for it - yes - on top of the wardrobe! This led to a whole new episode.

A brief aside from the story, I had been reading about Celtic ways and had come to a section on shape-shifting. To get an idea of shape-shifting the book suggested that you tried imitating your pets and seeing things through their eyes. So there I was on all fours, crawling around the floor, looking at everything from their level and point of view.

I started off by following Taffcat on his rounds. After having his afternoon nap (this bit I was good at), it was off to the kitchen to see what might be on offer. Off I trotted to the kitchen along with Taffcat, much to Taffy's bemusement and then, putting on my best duck voice, I started quacking along with him. Taffy, seeing me on the same level as him, wasn't sure where to direct his best quack. After a bit of confused quacking i.e. Taffcat quack, followed by me quacking, I eventually abandoned my shape-shifting for the day and stood up and gave Taffcat his food.

Now Tillcat posed a whole new challenge as she had taken to sleeping in the spare room, as well as sleeping on top of the wardrobe. Thankfully, on the day I chose to shape-shift into a Tillcat, Tilly opted for her bedroom to sleep. Now this I could do; sleeping on a nice comfortable bed was something at which I was quite expert. However, Tilly being a Tillcat doesn't sleep on the bed in a normal way. Oh no! Tilly squeezes herself between two pillows and forms a Tillcat pillow sandwich. I was now committed to being a Tillcat and did my best to curl up Tilly style between the other two pillows. So there I was sandwiched between two pillows asleep next to Tilly. I woke up stiff two hours later, not quite sure what I was doing!

The Celtic Holy Grail Quest

Seriously though, as mentioned in previous chapters, shape-shifting into an animal was an ancient Druid practice. They would enter shamanic trances and assume the form of their totemic animal for spirit journeys to the Celtic underworld. In my search for the Grail I have tried to attune myself to animals, for they can guide you across the boundary between the corporeal and the spirit world. When out walking keep a look out for animals and see where they go, for they could lead you to the Celtic underworld. White hares are well known to be able to bridge the gaps between worlds. Cats of course have long been associated with other worlds, in particular as witches' familiars, which have more ancient Druid roots. Back to feeding Tilly on top of the wardrobe. Having gained an insight into our two cats' minds, I now was witness to an exemplary display of cat psychology, as seen from their point of view. The first time we fed Tilly on top of the wardrobe, neither of the cats was aware of the new location for Tilly's food. I gave Taffy a mid morning snack of ham and he enjoyed it so much that he decided to have a post-snack snack. So off he jumped onto the counter to snack on Tilly's breakfast. (Tilly does not normally eat her breakfast until later in the day and then not all of it). He was totally dismayed when he found that Tilly's breakfast was not there! Where had it gone?

Now Taffy has a highly sensitive Taff-snack sniffer and he traced the smell of Tuna to our bedroom.

David Stocks

However on arrival in the bedroom, he could not locate the tuna and he sat on the windowsill puzzled.

Tilly then got up from her bedroom and trotted downstairs. Sherlock Taffy, now in detective mode, crept downstairs behind Tilly, hoping to follow her to the new location of Tilly's food. Tilly, having now accepted the fact that Taffy got all of her food from the counter, went out hunting. Taffy, on trail of Tilly's secret stash of Tuna, followed Tilly out of the cat flap.

Magpie Till and Taff Shady (legends in the cat underworld) ventured out in search of food. After a prolonged period of time, Taffy returned home, having failed to find Tilly's new tuna supply. He crept upstairs and went back into the bedroom, where he had first scented the tuna.

Will Taffy locate the Tuna? If so will he attempt the north face of the wardrobe in a valiant effort to reach the tuna? Only time will tell.

Taffy promptly fell asleep on the bed, exhausted from his tuna detective work. Meanwhile Tilly returned back to base and, opting for her high sleeping place, leapt to the top of the wardrobe where much to her delight she found the tuna. Having not eaten for some considerable period of time, Tilly wolfed the tuna down. Taffy, on hearing the frenzied feeding perked his ears up, but alas, having exhausted himself on his hunt for tuna,

The Celtic Holy Grail Quest

could not quite rouse himself from his sleep. Tilly finished off her tuna in peace and all was well with the world.

The cats have been of immense value to me during my bouts of depression, especially Taffy who is very intuitive and reads my moods well. Any time I am feeling low, Taffy snuggles up to me and purrs away and I find him very therapeutic and uplifting.

For those of you who do not have so much contact with the animal world, try to tune in to the way of animals. There is a lot more about them than modern man understands, lost knowledge long forgotten. We need to be more in tune with nature and uncover her secrets. What nature instils in me is peace and tranquillity and I go to her much as a child goes to its mother.

David Stocks

Chapter 41 The incident of the taxis in the rain

So taken were we with the Lake District, that within a month we decided to return, this time for my birthday. This fell conveniently on a Sunday, in the tail end of October.

We set off from home early that Saturday, the day was overcast, but that didn't dampen our mood. We arrived late morning in the lakes and found our guest house, tucked off on a tiny little lane just out from the centre of Windermere. The drive up to the lodge was extremely steep and curved round sharply. We pulled up, tyres spinning and engine roaring, a sharp dash seeming the only way to make it up the challenging entrance. We were welcomed by the landlady, a very friendly woman, who showed us proudly to our room. It was full of character, with a magnificent four poster bed, hung with elegant linen curtains. What's more it had a sumptuous marble bathroom, with a sunken jacuzzi bath. On setting out again, we ordered a taxi for that evening, from one of a number of firms listed in the guest house. We wanted to make sure we made it in plenty of time for my birthday meal that Jules had booked at the Glass House restaurant in Ambleside.

We spent the day meandering around Ambleside, a beautiful little Lake District town. The Lake District is blessed with beauty, beauty of the hills and valleys, but even more so the inner beauty of the people, who are amongst the friendliest and

The Celtic Holy Grail Quest

kindest people in Britain. This was displayed in the cheery helpfulness we were greeted with in cafes and shops, an attitude that should be adopted more often elsewhere. On one such occasion, we purchased a pair of walking boots, the shopkeeper struck up conversation with us and lent us socks to try the boots on with. We joked about the darkening skies and the rain that was coming. Despite already only paying half price for the boots, he gave us a hefty discount on walking socks too, even though he didn't have to. On leaving we made a comment about traversing Kirkstone Pass to visit Kirkstone Inn again. The shopkeeper looked suitably impressed and it was with some reluctance that we admitted that we were going to make the ascent by car and not via the newly acquired footwear.

Having warmed ourselves with mulled wine at Kirkstone Inn, we ventured further afield in search of the Celtic Cumbrian roots.
Cumbria is not often remembered as the great Celtic kingdom it once was, that of Rheged, the capital of which was at Carlisle. It was one of the most powerful Celtic kingdoms at the time of the Roman retreat.

In search of this Celtic history we returned to Ambleside and journeyed out to Castlerigg, just outside Keswick. Castlerigg is one of Britain's oldest stone circles, dating back to approximately 3000 BC. A legacy of ancient Britons and the Celts followed. The stone circle lies on high open ground, framed by brooding lake district mountains, in a true amphitheatre of the gods. A total of thirty eight stones form an oval – it being not quite circular – which is thirty metres in diameter. Standing in the centre of these stones on that open hilltop, I could feel the Kingdom of Rheged calling me. The ancient wisdom hidden in these stones remains a secret. But, as with most stone circles, it could well have been part of a celestial observatory.

On our return from Castlerigg, we passed the location of Dunmai,l King of Cumbria in 945 AD. Dunmail Raise near Grasmere takes its name from a cairn built on top of Dunmail's body. Dunmail is a possible candidate for the Arthurian legend 'the once and future king.' It is said that following the battle some of Dunmail's warriors fled with the crown of Cumbria, escaping into the mountains to Grisedale Tarn. Here they threw it into the depths, where it would be safe until some future time when Dunmail would rise again and reclaim his crown. Each year the warriors are said to return and bring back the crown from the depths of the tarn. They would then carry it to the cairn where they struck it with their spears. A voice from the deep would reverberate, 'Not yet, not yet; wait awhile my warriors.'

We returned to our accommodation, for a night we were going to remember. A chain was to unfold that seemed to be totally out of our control. It was the night of the incident of the taxis. I shall replace the immortal king's words with: 'Not yet, not yet;

The Celtic Holy Grail Quest

wait a while my travellers.'

Before we even got to the taxi episode, things were already going awry. Having the luxury of a jacuzzi bath, we decided to be decadent and pour ourselves a glass of fine wine to enjoy in the bubbling waters of the bath. As it was my birthday, Jules made a point of running the bath and lighting candles ready for our relaxing dip. Ignoring the wide selection of bath essences, provided for use by the lodge, Jules decided to add her own herbal bubble bath to the water; her own special touch.

The bath being run, we switched on the jets and retired to the room, to watch the end of a TV programme, while sipping some wine. It was some while later when we eventually switched off the TV, undressed and made our way into the bathroom. With a gasp of anticipation of our candlelit soiree in the jacuzzi, we swung open the door to the bathroom. Oh for hindsight! On opening the bathroom, a wave of foam crashed down on us and washed into the room, drowning us in bubbles. The jacuzzi's air jets had created foam of gargantuan proportions. There was a reason for the guest house providing bath essences; they were of the non foaming variety, something we failed to take into account.

It took a long time to clear the bathroom, but fortified with wine and suffering from bouts of hysterical laughter, the job didn't seem such a chore. When we eventually relaxed into our non

David Stocks

foaming jacuzzi, we sipped wine while the jets massaged our bodies, soothing us and revitalising us ready for our evening out.

Ten minutes early, we went down to reception to wait for our taxi. After a prolonged wait, no sign of the taxi, so we ventured out into the rain to see if it was outside. Ten minutes later, the taxi still hadn't appeared and wet and annoyed we phoned the taxi firm to see what was going on. The lady on reception was somewhat abrupt with Jules, saying, 'If you have not got the courtesy to be at the pickup point on time, the taxi will not wait for you.' She reluctantly agreed to send another taxi.

Again we waited, the rain now absolutely pouring down. Jules stayed inside, while I kept dashing outside to see if the taxi was there. It was after quite some time, that I noticed a path going down from the front of the property. I only took note of it when I saw another guest returning up it. I ventured down and emerged onto a road, the rain now sheeting down. To my delight, out of the murkiness I saw the friendly orange glow of a taxi sign, on a cab that had just pulled up. Quickly I opened the door to the taxi and told the driver to hold on while I fetched Jules from the guest house. He seemed a pleasant soul and waited while I returned to the lodge. Dashing up the steps and along the path, I flung open the door and called to Jules to come quickly as our taxi had finally arrived.

The Celtic Holy Grail Quest

As we dashed outside I noticed another couple in reception, one of whom was the man I had seen coming up the path earlier. A fact that shall become relevant later in this tale.

We dived in the cab and were quickly whisked off towards our destination. By this time I was absolutely drenched, soaked through to the skin, my clothes clinging to me in a sodden embrace. Jules, whose patience had been pushed to the limit, was now livid at the whole episode. Anger, that had been sparked by the rudeness of the taxi coordinator and long waits in the rain, was further fuelled by her concern that we would be late for my birthday meal. The poor taxi driver, who was seemingly quiet and polite, was now on the receiving end of the following tirade.

'I hope my boyfriend doesn't come down with a fever, he's soaked through and he's only just got over a virus! Our taxi should have been here over half an hour ago and we shall be late for our meal!'

The taxi driver, ever the gentle soul, apologised profusely and assured us that this didn't normally happen with their taxi firm. He then pulled up at Francine's, a restaurant in Windermere, notifying us of our arrival. This left us flabbergasted.

'Francine's,' cried Jules with her hands on her hips and lips tightly pursed, 'But we booked to go to the Glass House!'

David Stocks

The taxi driver, at a loss, apologised once again and got straight on to the radio to the taxi station. He told the girl that we had booked to go to the Glass House, but she replied that no it was definitely Francine's that we had booked.

This was all too much for Jules. 'Well I never, the little liar, not only was she rude to me, the taxi half an hour late, but she also got the destination wrong!' (Big sigh) 'I understand it's not your fault, but I am totally exasperated with this firm!'

'I am really sorry,' the taxi driver replied. 'I've never known this happen before, she is normally very efficient. I will take you to the Glass House straight away'.

The rest of the journey to the Glass House in Ambleside passed in a frosty silence, with only a few polite comments from the driver. On arrival the rain was still bucketing down and the driver came round and opened the door for us. He then offered to escort Jules to the door under his umbrella, a nicer more chivalrous taxi driver you could not hope to meet. I commented quietly to the driver, 'I am very disappointed with your taxi firm and the rudeness that has been shown to Jules, but I don't hold you responsible as you have been very kind and efficient.'

He offered to pick us up later, to which I replied, 'Under no circumstances do we ever want to use

The Celtic Holy Grail Quest

your firm again!'

As a final peace offering before we left, he knocked a few pounds off the taxi fare.

We entered the Glass House, an oasis of warmth and light, on that cold rainy night. The staff greeted us like long lost friends, even though we had only eaten there once before and were also late. Quickly they escorted us to a cosy candlelit table, in the corner of the restaurant and presented us with their superb menu. The taxi ordeal was soon forgotten, as we dined like kings on fabulous food and wine. Our repast was interrupted when halfway through the main course, a nervous looking waitress approached us. She handed us a card for a taxi firm.

She then relayed a message. 'We have been asked to give you this card as apparently there has been some mix up with the taxi in which you arrived. It was not actually the firm you originally booked with. They asked me to pass this card on, so you can book a return trip with them if you want to.'

We both looked at each other sheepishly and thanked her. It slowly became apparent to us what must have happened. The taxi we originally booked had let us down, or (more likely) turned up at the front path of the guest house, that we didn't know existed. After waiting what seemed like an eternity for our taxi, I had found the front path and upon exploring it, found it led to a road on which another taxi had pulled up outside. Excitedly I had grabbed the taxi, having first gone back to collect Jules. We now realised that the couple waiting in reception with us must have been the people who had actually booked this taxi, and we had hijacked it! Hence we were delivered to Francine's and not the Glass House. We had then proceeded to complain bitterly all the way. Through a series of misunderstandings, we had wreaked havoc, leaving a trail of people and taxis in our wake. We were now left with no option: We were duty bound to book a return trip with the taxi firm to whom earlier we had so bitterly complained.

Before the ground could swallow us up, the dessert arrived and I was in for a very pleasant surprise. My chocolate mousse came on an enormous porcelain plate. It had a candle in it and beautifully written in chocolate sauce around the rim of the plate was: 'Happy Birthday David.' It certainly was a birthday to remember. On finishing the dessert we plucked up the courage and booked a taxi. It arrived within a couple of minutes, before we could order a coffee. We paid the bill and were courteously escorted to our taxi, which was no less than a limousine! Rather than take offence at our earlier behaviour, the taxi firm were pulling out all the stops to impress us on our return journey. The limo must have been waiting outside for our call. So having stolen someone else's taxi and made false accusations to an undeserving taxi firm, we were driven back in

The Celtic Holy Grail Quest

style.

On return to the guest house, we relaxed in our four poster bed and drank the rest of our wine, bursting into fits of hysteria at the night's events. This brought repeated knocks at our door with requests for us to 'Keep the noise down.' We could only hope it wasn't the same people who had lost their taxi to us. Like thieves in the night, we stole their taxi and now had come back to haunt them.

At midnight Jules gave me some birthday presents, all beautifully wrapped and I opened them excitedly in our four poster bed. The whole night was memorable.

The next morning we fretted about going down to breakfast. We didn't want to chance an encounter with the other people of the taxi episode. We were prompted into action by a knock at our door 'Breakfast is being served,' pause, 'If you want it?'

We made our way down to breakfast with much trepidation. Much to our relief, our friends from the night before were not there and we enjoyed a fabulous breakfast. The landlady was as friendly as ever, giving us advice on where we could go that day and we left in good spirits.

I feel somewhat shameful of the incident now and if you happen to be reading this book, fellow travellers of the night, I apologise for acquiring a

David Stocks

taxi that was not rightfully ours. My apologies also extend to the taxi firms concerned.

Despite all our unintentionally disreputable behaviour and sequence of misunderstandings, the landlady made a big fuss of us and was constantly cheerful and helpful throughout. If she only knew the full story! We have not since returned to that guest house.

The Celtic Holy Grail Quest

Chapter 42 Dark Omens as the Banshee sings

On return from our trip to the lakes, we were filled with a primeval energy, a thirst for the outdoors and nature. With winter approaching, the days were now very short and because of work commitments, we were only able to venture outside at night. We took to walking the country lanes surrounding Stonnall each evening, when Jules returned from the office. Walking at night is a very profound experience and the solitude of our surroundings was blissful. It permeated the air, as we traversed ancient paths by starlight, peaceful and all encompassing. We felt at one with the world and could feel the Celtic otherworld calling us, the silvery glow of the twilight hours bringing the mystic otherworld within our reach.

It was while on these walks that we saw a shooting star make its fiery way across the skies, a stellar message from the Celtic gods. We followed its trail as it made its way over a hilltop on which a lone tree stood. I was reminded of the shooting star I had seen at Carcassonne; I hoped it would bring me luck on my quest for the Grail. Legends of fiery dragons had been born of meteor trails. It was a few nights before Samhain (Halloween) at around this time last year that I had journeyed deep beneath Rock Cemetery. I had felt a connection with the Celtic underworld, a shift in the air resonated with underworld frequencies, inviting me to return to that realm to seek

David Stocks

inspiration. So on the night of Samhain, we set out on our journey to the top of Grove Hill, over which the shooting star had cast its light.

The evening was moody; dark clouds bubbled in the sky like the contents of a witch's cauldron. The night air was surprisingly still, but it oozed tension; could this be the calm before the storm? Silently we trod along paths of old, lost in our own thoughts. In our hands we held lanterns, Halloween lanterns from Jules' childhood, in the guise of skulls. We made our way to the base of the hill, the lone tree on top silhouetted black against the night sky. The trunk and branches stretched upwards, like a skeletal hand erupting from the ground below.

The tree was ancient and steeped in history; legend has it that Romans were hanged from its branches on their arrival in this Celtic land and that the hill was an ancient burial site. As we ascended the hill, the wind picked up and tried to force us back down its eerie slopes. Leaning into the wind, so that our bodies were almost parallel to the hill, we pushed on upwards, defying the elements and the forces of Mother Nature. Legs aching and out of breath, we finally made it to the summit of the hill. A gale was now howling around us. From the complete calm of the valley, an unknown force had been summoned and cast its mighty hand against us.

Sheltering against the tree, in the lee of the wind,

The Celtic Holy Grail Quest

the gale howled through the branches and around its base. It shrieked, like an all despairing wail, assailing us from both sides. It was the cry of the banshee, foretelling a death soon to come. The underworld was reaching out to claim its latest soul in a deathly embrace. My imagination propelled me down towards the denizens below.

Dirt blew up from the barren hilltop and swirled around like spirits of the dead, screaming their message of doom, of fear and dread. The cold wind tore through our clothing, its icy fingers clenching our hearts, trying to stop their beats. All my years of depression came crashing down on me and I felt myself drowning in a sea of sorrow. My voyage into the underworld that night was not in search of the Grail. It was a voyage into the heart of my misery, depression and self loathing. I looked in on myself and I found myself wanting. I saw what I had become, a moody person, not at rest with myself and my spirit within. I felt I had under achieved, I was of no value as a person and with that I cried. My grief flooded out from me, tears like acid dropped into the soil - I did not like being me. I felt life's energy drain from within; with the tears leaked my vitality and so I died.
I died in my mind that night. For years I had been suffering from self loathing and pity. High up on that hill I let it all out.

I fell into a void. Time had no meaning here, space was an illusion, there was no up, no down, no backwards, no forwards. I lost myself in that void, not black, not white, but a grey neutral zone, my mind searching for a home. I was a rag doll, collapsed against that lone tree. I was numb. I was nothing.

I was a tiny particle in an infinitesimal space, sparked into existence and then expanded bigger and bigger, like the birth of the universe, the big bang. Brighter and brighter it shone, casting its radiance upon my soul, anointing me with its holy glow. I felt warmth course back through my body and with a jolt neurons fired within my brain. On that lonely hilltop, I was reborn.

Dust from centuries of heartache cracked from my eyes, opening to a new different world from the one I had just left. Down on my knees I cast my eyes upwards and looked into the face of an angel. My guardian angel. Jules leaned over me, her head covered by a hood, with the silvery disc of the moon behind it framing her in a spectral fantasy, shimmering like a celestial halo. A tear dropped from her left eye and sparkled like a diamond as it fell in slow motion to alight in my right eye, flooding me with its light. Then a smile spread across my angel's face and I felt myself embraced in her wings.

We stayed interlaced, two figures alone on a hill, a tree standing guard over its earthen children. My mind had taken a flight of fancy. Or had it? Who knows? I had released my sorrows and was born anew.

The Celtic Holy Grail Quest

Twice reborn, just one more battle with my inner demons awaited me, before I could be finally released from their shackles and live free from torment.

Chapter 43 Alternative medicine and a new future

Having now lived at Jules' house for a long time, we decided that I should make it official and move in permanently. Part of this process was changing my doctor. As I now lived in Stonnall with Jules, I registered with Jules' doctor in the nearby town of Aldridge.

After my experience on Grove hill, I began to have severe mood dips, during which time a dark desperation engulfed me. After completing a new patient health check, I arranged an appointment with Jules' doctor for the following day, as a matter of urgency.

Having appraised my condition, he could see that the lows I was hitting were having a significant effect on my mental health and he referred me to the crisis team.

I met with the crisis team later that day; it being Friday I couldn't get to see a psychiatric doctor and so I was put on emergency medication over the weekend. The team were very supportive and went out of their way to help me.

I saw the team two more times over the weekend, during which time I got talking to one of the psychiatric nurses about alternative medicine. It turned out that he was skilled in acupuncture,

The Celtic Holy Grail Quest

something I had been thinking about having for some time. He was a great guy and we chatted about things in general, rather than my mental problems. This has always been my preferred way of dealing with depression, distraction being the best form of prevention. I find if you keep the mind busy, you don't have time to become depressed. Having shown my enthusiasm for acupuncture he agreed to come round on Tuesday and perform it on me.

I had also been researching alternative medicines on the Internet and had found a site offering herbal remedies from Tibet, an institute backed by the Dalai Lama. Having found his book 'The Art of Happiness' so successful in getting me through a depressive period in the past, I was keen to try the herbal remedies on offer. There was no remedy specific to depression, but there was one that helped rejuvenate the body and help protect the mind against mental problems. This was aptly named 'The elixir of rejuvenation.'

I began taking this Tibetan remedy at the start of the waxing of the moon, as instructed on the packet. From there onwards I drank the elixir dissolved in hot water first thing each morning, followed by a light stint of exercise (for me this was press-ups). I found this routine each morning energised me and equipped my body and mind with the vital force I needed to tackle each day.

On Monday the doctor came out to see me,

accompanied by two members of the crisis team. It so happened that one of the cats had caught a mouse that weekend that had escaped somewhere in the house, its exact whereabouts unknown. Talking with Jules, we envisaged the embarrassing scenario of the mouse scuttling across the room while the doctor was present, shortly to be followed by a cat in hot pursuit. However, it didn't happen quite like that. Oh no!

It was when I was in deep discussion with the doctor about my ebbing mental health, that Taffy took centre stage. Taffy had spotted the mouse moving in the curtains next to the tv. He then proceeded to pursue the mouse by leaping onto the tv with a loud clatter. Taffy, then somewhat off balance, stood precariously on top of the tv, teetering for a few anxious seconds until the law of gravity took hold. At this point, with ponderous inevitability, he slid unceremoniously down the back of the tv. All of his claws scratched at the plastic as he made his inglorious exit, culminating with a huge crash as he landed in a heap in amongst the cables.

The room went deathly silent; even Taffy in his shock didn't move. Then everybody burst out laughing at the whole incident which had been so ridiculous and amusing. Poor Taffy picked himself up, dusted himself down and slunk into another room. It took a while for the laughter to die down, but it was like a breath of fresh air, discharging the tension that had been present in the atmosphere.

The Celtic Holy Grail Quest

Laughter is good for the soul and all doctors should prescribe it as a tonic. Taffy, however, his pride in tatters, was not to be seen again for quite some time.

I last saw the mouse scuttling across the top of the curtain pole – I could have sworn it was laughing to itself – it was a real ginger Tom and Jerry episode.

The doctor eventually recovered the situation and we agreed that medication was probably not the best solution to my problems, as it had not had much effect on my illness in the past. He told me to use all the techniques I was currently using i.e. exercise, fresh air, keeping busy and suggested that we review it at the end of the week.

I had my acupuncture the next day which involved the careful placement of five needles into each ear. The effect was astounding. On the placement of the first needle, I went light headed and after they were all in place I started to float away. My mind became disconnected from my body and I felt I was hovering a few feet away. I relaxed for about twenty minutes after the needles were inserted, before they were removed again. I floated off, like a fluffy cloud in a blue sky, drifting over an aquamarine sea. I felt like an angel.

I was astounded by the effects of acupuncture, having never had it before. The treatment gave me an overall feeling of calmness that lasted well into the next day and I would recommend it to anyone.

I was reminded of my earlier thoughts, on the strategic placement of stones and trees along ley lines, akin to acupuncture for Mother Earth. Could we heal the planet by restoring ancient monuments and groves and realigning the planet's nervous system, or through the modern practice of Geomancy, using iron bars sunken into the ground?

The Celts venerated the Sky Father, Lugh, and the Earth Mother, Don. When I had acupuncture I became detached from my body. Thus I was in touch with both the Sky Father and Earth Mother at once. Perhaps through the placement of monuments, the Celts were trying to harmonize the Sky Father and Earth Mother?

The Celtic Holy Grail Quest

Chapter 44 Angels sing on Castle Ring

With my continuing descent into depression, Jules stayed at home to keep me company and we went walking each morning. Jules had come to me as an angel in my dreams and to me she was my guardian angel, come to heal me.

The day after the treatment, Jules suggested that we go for a walk on Cannock Chase. On our way there we decided to try and find Castle Ring ancient monument. Try as we might, we couldn't locate it and ended up parking outside the Windmill pub on Gentleshaw Common. From here we walked along narrow paths, through groves of trees and eventually out onto an exposed hilltop. The valley spread out majestically below us. From this sweeping vista we returned to the woods and completed a circuit, to return us back to the pub. Along the way Jules plucked a twig from a tree and held it in her left hand, as a guide for our return journey. It was a habit of Jules' to pick up a twig when out walking and would often lead her safely to her destination.

Encouraged by our success with the stick, Jules suggested that I hold it in the car while she drove, and we continued our search for Castle Ring. I took the stick, again in my left hand, and suggested turns as she drove. After a few turns and two or three minutes' drive, we ended up at Castle Ring. I have since read that the Celts are known to ask trees for a stick when they are out in

David Stocks

the woods. If the trees accept the request, they can break a stick off and use it as a wand (extension of the body) when they are out walking. The left hand is supposed to have psychic powers. We both followed intuition when tracing our routes; how much the stick had to do with it, I don't know? I do however know that in a later walk we made from Castle Ring, we could certainly have done with some intuition.

Castle Ring turned out to be an ancient fort. The ring is an Iron Age hill fort, a giant circular enclosure, made up of steep earthen mounds running right around the circumference. Time and erosion had worn it down and it had lost some of its stature that it had when the Celts were there. It was still impressive though. Some of the banks still stood four metres tall and the sheer scale of the site was awesome.

At the time of the Celts the whole perimeter of the circle would have been topped by wooden staves, with massive wooden gates being the only way in. People would have lived within the enclosure, in large circular thatched huts, with peat fires for cooking and eating.

We were as angels together, just for that moment in time, the skies clear, and a wind making the trees sing.

    Oh Castle Ring,
    Standing proud on top of the world,

The Celtic Holy Grail Quest

Angels sing,
Dancing with joy, wings unfurled.

A hilltop fort,
Through millennium, not forgotten,
A circular time-warp,
How many people here, have trodden.

Roman soldiers fall,
Crushed against its mighty bastions,
Celtic heroes stand tall,
Defying the giant Roman legions.

Lightly we tread,
Around this historic loop,
Unravelling the thread,
In its cosmic soup.

Crossing the threshold,
Into the ring's earthen heart,
We embrace in a hold,
Back in time we dart.

All is silent,
Two thousand years, stripped bare,
Time is pliant,
For travellers, who dare.

Around the rim,
A reindeer runs wild,
Circling in,
Sweet nature's child.

David Stocks

The mighty stag,
With antlers held proud,
Through a time lag,
Like a storm cloud.

Lightning for antlers,
Hooves sounding thunder,
The whole ring shudders,
And we're cast asunder.

The mighty reindeer,
Breaks into our realm,
And gallops clear,
Through ash and through elm.

Into the distance,
Along paths rarely trodden,
Swallowed in an instance,
To follow, we are bidden.

Lost in time, cast adrift with our thoughts, we stood staring along the track left by the Lord of Castle Ring. Entranced we strode out, hands clasped together, tracing the route left by that noble creature. It was not a vision, for the deer was plainly real, but it left behind an air of mystery.

Its trail disappeared, deep into the woods, weaving a secret path into a dell. We followed the meandering path down and up a steep sided slope, where it joined a broad track heading for a ridge. Onwards and upwards we climbed, to where we knew not? A final rise exited onto a

The Celtic Holy Grail Quest

clearing. From here a thin track could be seen, snaking over the other side of the ridge. Taking this track we went in search of the forest king.

The path became steep and rugged, our footing unsure, but with many a stumble we wended our way down. Abruptly a small ravine opened up before us and before I could stop I launched into the air careering over the chasm. The wind rushed through my hair and everything slowed down. I could make out a squirrel running up a tree, smell fresh pine in the air, see the ripples in the water below, and hear birds singing. Then with a thud, my feet struck the marshy bank on the opposite side and I fell to the ground. The drop must have been a good ten feet, but the soft ground had cushioned my fall and I got up somewhat dazed but safe and sound.
Jules thankfully had managed to stop in time, but we now had the problem of getting her to the other bank. Slowly I encouraged her to climb down carefully, which she did bravely, but the slope was steep and muddy and she was soon sliding on her backside down to the bottom. Again the ground was marshy when she hit the bottom and she came to an abrupt halt with a squelch. Unhurt by her tumble, Jules crossed the stream on a series of stepping stones, swift water washing over her boots. She was now covered in mud, twigs and leaves entangled in her braids. The Jules that had started the descent down the ravine and the Jules that emerged on the other side were two totally different beings. For Jules was now a swamp

David Stocks

monster!

We cleaned Jules up as best we could and then examined the terrain ahead. All the tracks had disappeared, the woodland deeply covered by dense undergrowth and logs. Totally disorientated we had to head blindly out. Keeping as best we could on a straight line, we eventually emerged on a track. We followed this upwards trying to find Castle Ring, which was on high ground. We stumbled upon a small glade. The glade was home to an ancient oak tree that reminded me very much of the Major Oak in Sherwood Forest. This was the old man of the forest and it was to him the deer had led us. Its trunk was massive in circumference and gnarled with age and time, wrinkled like an old man's skin. The glade was absolutely tranquil. Gently we placed our hands on the tree and prayed to the Celtic gods to help us with our future. A feeling of warmth and peace spread through us and we stayed like that for some time, embracing the tree, embracing time.

Having paid homage to the venerable tree, we left that peaceful glade in search of our way back. We crossed little wooden bridges over streams, crested ridges and even passed a tiny wooden hut, of the type witches would dwell in.

We were lost, but calm inside after our encounter with the old man of the forest. We never doubted that we would find our way back.

The Celtic Holy Grail Quest

After about an hour's hike we reached the sanctuary of a road, where parked at the side we found two workman in a truck. Having now no idea where we were, we asked the men for directions to Castle Ring. This amused them greatly, as we were obviously nowhere near the ancient monument and it took much scratching of heads before they pointed across the road in the vague direction they thought it must be.

Crossing the road we took their advice and found a track that roughly followed that direction. Sometime later we came to a small lake and spied in the distance a large sawmill. We had seen buildings of similar ilk from on top of Castle Ring and decided this must be the direction we had to go. The sawmill turned out to be huge in size and it was only after skirting it for quite some time that Jules decided to ask some horse riders the way. They pointed back to the lake and told us to follow the track up from there and turn left when we reached the road. This we did and after three hours lost in the forest we found our way back to the car park at Castle Ring.

We felt we had been tested, but not found wanting and received the blessing of the old man of the forest as a reward.

On another visit to Castle Ring, we stayed within a safe distance of the hill fort and were wandering through the forest when a dog came bounding up to us. The dog was playful and we patted its head joyfully. We then heard a woman calling the dog back, as she approached us from further down the trail. She had another dog on a lead.

She then said the memorable words, 'This one's alright, it's just eaten some horse shit.'

We smiled at her, trying to control our laughter and commented on the beautiful morning and complemented her on her lovely dogs.

Our walk continued back to the foot of Castle Ring, the slopes glistening white with crystalline frost in the morning sunlight. Jules skittered to the top of the slope, fresh with the joys of spring and I took a photo of her. High on that circle of light, a beautiful maiden stood tall.

From behind me I heard a familiar voice, asking: 'Would you like me to take a picture of you both?'

It was the friendly lady with her two dogs. We thanked her and said, 'Yes, that would be lovely.'

I handed her the camera and ran up the hill to join Jules. We stood together, snuggled into one another, while the tranquillity of that special place washed over us.

Retrieving the camera, we thanked her again and she smiled, pleased to have been of help. We felt we had made a new friend and parting she said, 'See you again.'

The Celtic Holy Grail Quest

The picture is one we will treasure forever; in it we are as one, at peace, up high on God's own garden. Whether we will see her again, I don't know, but something makes me think we will.

On our only trip to Castle Ring at night, the whole place was spookily silent. Ascending to the top of the ring, we felt an ethereal presence; a deep chill pervaded the air. As we walked round, the bright points of starlight closed in on us and we sensed a menace in the air. It was as if we were intruding where we were not wanted.

We circumnavigated the ring, the stars spinning high up around us. Every step brought further feelings of foreboding. Three quarters of the way round, our unease was beginning to shake us and we had quickened the pace. We made haste back towards the car park. It was then that we noticed a strange white light on the opposite rim of the ring. The light bobbed there for a few moments and we assumed it was either a bike or a walker with a torch. The light then began to descend towards the centre of the ring, rather than follow the path around the ring's perimeter. It flickered and bobbed from side to side as it made its way down and, unlike a walker or a cyclist, it moved erratically. Sometimes it would move inwards at speed, but then drift back slowly, almost as if it was scenting something. We began to feel nervous, and fearing we were the prey that it was hunting, we quickened our pace still more.

Sensing this, the light moved from the distance, shimmering out of focus, heading in a direct line for us. It looked to be moving slowly, but this was deceptive, as it soon made ground on us, as if bounding in giant steps. Now full of fear, we made our final flight and broke into a run. Slipping on damp earth we stumbled down the steps from the ring and out into the car park. Looking back we saw the light hovering on the edge of the ring and then it disappeared. We knew not what it was? Whatever it was, we would not like to venture out there again in the pitch black of night. We have not returned to Castle Ring at night since.

Chapter 45 Psychic Power and Earth Energy

Everything I do I believe has a reason and is interconnected with past and future events. The course of my life is like a stream, starting with little rivulets of interspersed events that join together in a stream. The stream follows the rich pattern of life; meandering it snakes it way through life until it empties out into a lake of opportunity.

From this lake, infinitesimal possibilities spring. One such opportunity, presented to us as a realisation of a dream, was to found a new company. As part of the implementation stage, we needed to get organised and with this in mind I went into town to get stationery and files etc.

Having not much money at this point in our lives (this is an understatement), I made a special effort

The Celtic Holy Grail Quest

to shop around for the best deals. This bore fruit when I found a discount shop that specialised in books, stationery and art materials etc. While acquiring our much needed office supplies, I discovered a vastly reduced dowsing kit, by Uri Gellar. Uri Gellar is one of the most famous modern day psychics; while some may question his methods, he has astounded many with his apparent psychic ability. The kit included a workbook, a crystal pendulum and two dowsing rods. As previously mentioned, I was intrigued by dowsing and also felt an affinity with quartz, the piezoelectricity features of which is used in a clock's electronics. Perhaps it made the universe tick? I left the shop with a well equipped office – paper, pens, files, binders – oh, and one dowsing kit. Well, no office should be without one!

I returned home and Jules was soon busy organising the files and I was kept occupied with other aspects of starting up a business. It was not until a few days later, that our attention was drawn to the dowsing kit.

I was busy making our evening meal, when Jules came down from the office, tired and feeling a bit under the weather after a hectic day's work. I suggested that she sat down and had a look at the dowsing kit.

Jules settled down and was soon engrossed in the book and she gave a yelp of delight when she discovered the pendulum.

David Stocks

'I used to do this years ago,' she exclaimed. 'I used a cotton thread and a key at the time. I had no idea that it was a recognised dowsing method.'

She then proceeded to tell me how the pendulum works. You hold it absolutely still in front of you and then ask it a question. The pendulum will then swing in a particular direction of its own accord. For example, for the answer 'yes' it will swing in a circle either clockwise or anticlockwise and for the answer 'no' it will swing from side to side either from left to right or diagonally.

Now all I had to do was go through the potential lottery numbers and ask the pendulum 'yes' or 'no,' whether the number was going to turn up that week.
But prior to my get-rich-quick scheme, I asked Jules to demonstrate the pendulum. The room was tranquil, lit by candles, with gentle Celtic music playing in the background. Jules sat crossed legged in front of the fire, breathed in and composed herself. Reaching deep inside, she found a point of inner calm. Extending the pendulum in front of her so that there was no movement, she addressed it.
'Will our business succeed?' This induced the pendulum to swing in an anticlockwise direction, much to my relief!
Jules then urged me to ask the pendulum a question. I asked it, 'Does Jules love me?' To my even greater relief, the pendulum spun clockwise

The Celtic Holy Grail Quest

with great earnest. It was a question to which I hoped I knew the answer, but it was still a relief when the pendulum confirmed it.

After asking a number of other questions and receiving a 'yes' or 'no' response, we decided to give the copper dowsing rods a try.

Jules held these in the manner specified in the accompanying book, having never dowsed with rods before, and tried to find water. When holding rods out in front of you, they should twitch in the presence of water. Leaving nothing to chance, we decided to dowse the sink. This produced a dramatic result, but not one that we expected. The rods didn't twitch but Taffy went mental, jumping up at the sink as if he was trying to block our attempts at dowsing.

I strongly believe that animals have a sixth sense and if Taffy was not comfortable with us dowsing, then we had better stop.

Luckily for the national lottery, that put a stop to our dabbling with dowsing for that evening.

Over the course of the next few days we asked the dowsing pendulum some further questions, but nothing of significance. We did consider dowsing for concealed treasure, as the previous owner was known to have money, and we wondered whether he might have stashed some somewhere in the house!

The whole psychic thing came to a head one night, when after returning from a night out, we opened the door and were both hit by dizziness. This dizziness stayed with us all that night and into the next day. There was no reason for this, no gas leaks or abnormal weather conditions, but it only affected us in the house. This culminated with me asking the pendulum one final question, 'Is this house located on a place of power?' The pendulum responded by spinning so fast it nearly left Jules' hand. The answer was a resounding 'yes!'

We have not since used the dowsing kit and unfortunately didn't exploit the potential for winning the lottery. One thing on which I have had several wins since, although unfortunately not amounting to vast sums of money, is scratch cards. Jules' mum, Margaret, very generously buys them for Jules and me. On these I am a regular winner, but only on the 'Lucky Leprechauns.' This I put down to the luck of the Irish, their Celtic roots and the Irish Jig that I perform before revealing the card. It works nearly every time!

I would like to share with you one last instance concerning lucky omens. Quite some time after writing this chapter, Jules and I invited our parents round to watch the Grand National. My mother bet on Silver Birch, a tree she loves and one with Celtic connections that I have discussed. Ten minutes prior to the race Tilly climbed right up to the top of a Silver Birch in our back garden. We saw this as a good omen and Silver Birch subsequently romped home first.

The Celtic Holy Grail Quest

Chapter 46 Spidy goes to Wolverhampton

I have mentioned Jules' Alfa Romeo Spider in previous chapters, but I have not yet revealed its full character. Jules nicknamed her Alfa 'Spidy' and says that he is a typical Italian male, full of good looks and charisma, but with an Italian temperament to match. No truer words could be spoken, and with this in mind I have decided to dedicate an entire chapter to this cheeky little Italian car and in particular, one incident.

Our lives by this stage had become somewhat surreal and now the psychic phenomena was spreading to Jules' car. As demonstrated in this chapter, the intuitive link between mankind and nature had acquired a more modern counterpart, for as this chapter unfolds you will see what uncanny characteristics a car can display. I still strongly believe that we should live more in harmony with nature and use of automobiles should be kept to a minimum. But you cannot help but smile when you read about Spidy and it is to make you smile that I have written this chapter. A lot more wisdom can be gleaned from this incident; stay attuned for all will be revealed.

Spidy has many little quirks and likes to engage us in his automotive games. As with everything in our lives, he is far from a normal car. He has a list of little tricks he likes to play on us. One of his favourites is refusing to start, or worse still, stalling at a junction and then refusing to start. The only way round it, is to leave him for twenty minutes or more and then try starting him again. Then if he deigns it appropriate and has received the respect such a thoroughbred Italian car deserves, he will start. Another of his favourite tricks is to refuse to lock. On pressing the locking mechanism on the key fob, the lock buttons will go down and then pop immediately back up. Usually if you try for a while it will eventually lock. This locking problem was intermittent and didn't happen too often.

Following our discovery of Castle Ring, our little Italian friend started playing up more and more. At first it was the engine, refusing to be started, but he then got obsessed with refusing to lock. It got to a point that every time we drove it, we would get out of the car and Spidy just would not lock. We tried various techniques to try and combat Spidy's electronic psychological problems. These included:-

- Starting the engine, stopping it and locking him again.
- Opening the door, zapping him with the key fob (which would cause the alarm mechanism to bip), closing the door and zapping him again.
- Manually locking him with the key. The lock buttons on the door would still pop up, but you could sometimes overcome this by keeping the key turned.
- Unlocking, opening, closing and relocking the boot, then zapping him.

The Celtic Holy Grail Quest

- In one extreme event, inserting the radio, locking him, unlocking him, removing the radio and locking him again.

We tried all sorts of tricks to try and out-psyche his little electromotive brain. Whatever we tried would not work more than once however. There was no pattern or logic that we could follow.

The locking problem continued to get worse, until one day he started to refuse to unlock as well. We filled up with petrol and when I returned from paying, I could not get back in. Jules was in the car waiting to drive away, but try as I might, I could not get the door open. Jules tried opening it and unlocking him from the inside, but still no success. Spidy was definitely in a mood and did not want me back in the car. Eventually we had to admit defeat and I resorted to climbing in across the driver's seat to reach the passenger seat. I don't know what the petrol station attendants thought; the video of our activities is probably being mulled over by the police as I write this. On returning home we eventually managed to force open the door, with Jules tugging at the handle from the outside and me pushing from the inside. That was the last straw, Spidy was grounded! We used my car for the next week.

Now as you can see, this car has a real personality. Spidy did not like being grounded at all. He sat on the drive and gathered grime from the dank days we were having. He looked most forlorn; I know it sounds strange, but if a car can sulk, Spidy certainly sulked. It was when we left the house one day that Spidy finally gave in, and with a flash of his lights the door locks popped open. I know it is hard to believe, but we did not touch the key fob at all and Spidy literally decided to open for us. It was a plea from the heart, his little engine was racing, and he wanted to be back on the road.

We decided to give him another chance and drove out with him again. But alas, Spidy was still his old self and on arrival at our destination, we could not open the doors again. It was with a lot of effort and much cursing from Jules which she did in Italian - 'Santa Maria, Mama Mia!' - just to hammer the point home, that we finally opened the doors. We decided to keep using Spidy anyway, as we had now come to accept that we had to put up with his foibles.

I was asleep in bed late one night when the landline phone rang, followed by my mobile phone. I could not stir though and ignored them. Shortly afterwards, Jules came into the house cursing. She had been locked in Spidy and couldn't get out. She had phoned me to come outside and help her open Spidy. In the end she had resorted to climbing out of the driver's window in order to get out. This was all getting too much, we had to get Spidy into a garage, but we were low on funds and time. We had to find another solution. Eventually we discovered that we could open the doors by giving them a sharp punch with

The Celtic Holy Grail Quest

the base of our hands and so continued using him in his ever increasing fits of peak.

If what had already been happening wasn't enough, it finally all came to a head when we went to an important business meeting one morning. The meeting was in Hednesford and we arrived on time, with no problems from Spidy at all. We parked outside the place of our meeting and admired the beautiful sleek Aston Martin, whose owner we were going to see. I said to Jules, 'That's the car I'm going to have one day.' We both laughed and joked; one can but dream! After the meeting we came out and again admired the Aston Martin. We got into Spidy, but he wouldn't start. Now you may think I am paranoid, or maybe just delusional, but Spidy was definitely sulking. He didn't like the covetous looks we had been giving the Aston Martin. While we sat in the car park frustrated, not knowing what to do, we heard the Aston Martin burst into life, its exhaust growling with a throaty roar. We sat there distraught watching the Aston Martin sweep out of the gates, gleaming, pristine, but more to the point, moving!

We had no choice but to abandon Spidy and head off into Hednesford while we waited for him to come out of his sulk!

We walked the length of Hednesford High Street. On the way back we called in at the local bakery and bought some cakes for afternoon tea. They were very friendly in the shop and our spirits lifted. We returned to the car and low and behold, Spidy started first time. Heading back, I decided to try and take a short cut, having inherited my uncanny navigational skills from my father. We of course ended up lost. To foil our attempts at turning back, Spidy cut out again at a junction right on the brow of a hill. Try as we might, Spidy would not start again. We sat there helpless and watched a funeral cortège make its way sombrely past us on the road running across our junction. It seemed somewhat apt that Spidy should die at this point so sadly we gave him his last rights.

We now had no choice but to phone the RAC who promised to treat us as a priority, as we were blocking a junction. Happy in the knowledge that the RAC were on the way, we sat down and waited. Feeling a call of nature that became ever more urgent, I left Jules with the car and made my way across the road to Hednesford Community Hall which we had now discovered to be in Pye Green. On entering I was greeted by the friendly people working in the hall that day. I explained that I had broken down and asked if I could use their facilities. They smiled and said that they had seen us broken down and that it had happened to one of them not too long ago. They then went on to explain that it had taken five hours for them to be recovered. I told them, somewhat over confidently, that the RAC were coming to pick us up and that we had been deemed a priority as we were blocking a junction. They were only too glad

The Celtic Holy Grail Quest

to let me use the facilities and it was with relief that I returned to the car a few minutes later.

We had broken down at about 11.50 am and after waiting a while longer, Jules paid the community hall a visit. Having had tea and coffee at our meeting, it was lucky we had facilities in such close proximity! After about half an hour had passed and there was still no sign of the RAC, I attempted to push the car over the junction onto the road running across the top. I assured Jules that Spidy would not roll back over me and I should be able to push it, no problem. Flexing my herculean muscles, I braced myself against Spidy and told Jules to release the brake. I gave an almighty push and nothing happened. Again I asked Jules to release the brake; Jules assured me she had and again I gave a mighty push. This was it, man against machine, my raw animal power was going to be more than a match for this Italian motoring Goliath. I was, after all, David!

Spidy didn't budge! Sweating with exertion, I reluctantly asked Jules to apply the handbrake and somewhat red faced got back into the car - round one to Spidy.

The time ticked on and we kept trying the ignition to see if the car would start again, but Spidy was having none of it. Then, enter the scene, one man and his dog.

'Hi mate, having trouble?' he called across the

road.

'Just a bit,' I replied, 'Car won't start.' Then Jules called out (by this time totally exasperated), 'Don't buy Italian!'

'I'll help give you a push,' he called.

So there we were again, handbrake on, two men, one dog and a stubborn Alfa Romeo.

'Release the brake,' I cried. Pause. 'Release the brake,' I cried again.

'I have,' Jules replied. Muscles straining, I glanced over at my helper and he looked back at me, both of us sharing a look of disbelief. Surely two men were more than a match for this Italian machismo steel concoction of engine, wheels and bodywork?

The dog barked - not forgetting the dog of course! But despite the muscle power of two men and a dog, Spidy would not move - round two to Spidy.

Before leaving, the helpful passer-by suggested that we rolled the car back down the hill and pulled it out of the way of the junction. Easy we thought, gravity was now in our favour. Standing a safe distance behind the car, I called to Jules to take the handbrake off while I directed her.

Now there is one thing to know about modern cars, they rely on power steering and without the

The Celtic Holy Grail Quest

engine going there is no power steering. So there I am frantically signalling to Jules to turn the wheel, while the car was rapidly heading towards the curb. In a last ditch attempt to stop it, I ran to the side of the car and signalled Jules to stop. This she did and after many exclamations Jules explained that the steering wheel wouldn't turn. It was only then that we grasped the real significance of power steering.

Right, this was obviously a man's job, after all it is a man's world, men and motors. Out hopped Jules and into the cockpit I leapt. Spidy was no match for me and without releasing the handbrake I tugged the steering wheel round. With the steering on full lock, I released the handbrake, keeping my foot on the brake pedal to ease the car backwards.

The Alfa shot backwards; I don't know what the 0 to 60 time is for an Alfa Romeo Spider, but I am sure Spidy broke the fastest recorded time going backwards. My foot was pressed flat down on the brake pedal, but nothing was happening. I lurched forward in my seat as the car accelerated downhill and then slammed back against the seat as Spidy mounted the curb and stopped fast. I pulled the handbrake on, now a somewhat futile exercise, as the car was now jammed against the curb. Then cursing cars, engines and all things Italian, I ingloriously got out - round three to Spidy.

Nearly an hour had gone by and the RAC priority

recovery had still not turned up. We called the RAC and asked their mission control where exactly our friendly man in his fluorescent RAC jacket was. Mission control didn't have any record of our previous call and kindly asked us to hang on the line while they looked up our incident number. Ten minutes later and after being subjected to lots of piped music, the RAC operative remembered we were there and reported that the dedicated field operative was winging his way towards us any minute now. A further ten minutes passed and with all patience now totally exhausted we phoned the RAC yet again. We were then told that he was in fact still on another case and he would be on his way as soon as he had finished. We complained to the RAC, explaining in no uncertain terms that we had been waiting nearly an hour and a half and that the service levels in this country were appalling. We also stated that there was no way that we would be renewing our membership with the RAC. We hung up and realised we were in for a long wait. We now both felt very hungry and knew that it would be a long time until we got a meal. It was then that I remembered the cream cakes.

So there we were at the corner of the junction, with an Alpha Romeo Spider halfway up the curb and angled across the road, demolishing very moorish jam and cream cakes, icing powder decorating our noses and our suits. Yes, the very epitome of high powered executives! We were going places, or not, as the case was turning out

The Celtic Holy Grail Quest

to be. Just as we were finishing the cream cakes, the RAC called again and said that our long awaited field operative was nearly with us.
The funeral cortège that had passed us earlier when we broke down, now returned sombrely along the hilltop. We got back into the car again and tried the ignition one last time. Spidy started straight away. Great, we had broken all diplomatic relations with the RAC, insisted that they got to us urgently and now the Alpha was purring in a way any Italian sports car should. With a look in the rear view mirror, sure enough the RAC van was approaching. The van pulled up and the engineer got out. I looked sheepishly out of the window and explained to the engineer that we had been trying it constantly and it had only just started - round four to Spidy.

I still firmly believe that Italian family values had taken over and Spidy was only dutifully paying his respects.
To his credit, the engineer turned out to be as nice a guy as you could meet. He took in all we told him and agreed to escort us to the Alpha Garage in Wolverhampton. Off we drove and all was going well for about ten minutes, when Spidy slowed to a stop at another junction. The engineer got out and lifted the bonnet of our irascible Italian motor and started tweaking wires left right and centre. Try as he might he could not get the Alpha to start. He went into the van to study the Alpha's electrics on the computer. Emerging from the van he looked inside the boot in search of an alarm

override switch as it was the alarm system he had now diagnosed as the fault with the Spider. After much searching, he came out cursing the Alpha wiring diagram and comparing it to a plate of Italian spaghetti - round five to Spidy.

Right, Spidy had now declared war and left us with only one option! We called the Alpha Romeo Garage and told them that we were bringing Spidy back in shame. We sat in the RAC van's cab while the engineer hitched up Spidy and towed him back to the alpha garage in disgrace - round six to the RAC.

We arrived safely at our destination and thanked the engineer gratefully for bringing us and the Alpha to the garage. Jules was greeted by Adrian and Will of W.A.D. Alpha Romeo Engineering. They were long time friends of Jules and were soon chatting happily away with her. While Adrian worked on Spidy, Will chatted to Jules and me about Alfa Romeo cars. He told us an hilarious tale about an Alpha they had bought from a man who had gone bankrupt. Apparently the man had come in one day, along with both his wife and mistress. The car had been sold for cash for fifteen thousand pounds that was subsequently split between the three of them, each one therefore netting five thousand pounds!

Adrian eventually fixed Spidy, having diagnosed a problem with the wiring. He told us that the locking problem was due to a faulty cable inside the door.

The Celtic Holy Grail Quest

He showed us that the car could be locked by reaching in through the window and wiggling the driver's door handle backwards and forwards before pressing the zapper. The problem with this solution however, meant that the window would then be left open. He offered to spend another hour working on it to fix the door handle mechanism, but we were already grateful for what he had done and politely declined for the time being - round seven to W.A.D. Alpha Romeo.

On the way back we discussed the problem of locking the Alpha. I came up with the ingenious idea of the driver getting out first, while the passenger waited inside. Once the driver had got out, the passenger would then lean over and waggle the driver's door handle. The passenger would then get out and close the door, at which point the car could be zapped and it should lock ok. When we got back we tried this technique and to our amazement it worked first time. We were left with one last problem, however, what if there was no passenger? After a little thought, I came up with the following solution:-
The driver gets out and shuts the door, then opens the passenger door, leans over and wiggles the driver's door handle, closes the passenger door and then zaps the car. This we have since tried and it works perfectly. At the time of writing we have still got the better of Spidy and have no more problems - last and final round to Jules and Dave!

David Stocks

The psychological and analytical techniques that I used to combat the Spidy challenges in this chapter, have played a significant part in helping me to resolve the Grail mystery.

The Celtic Holy Grail Quest

Chapter 47 Not quite final destination

As a respite from the pressures of life, I went on a trip to Schladming (Austria) during the post Christmas to New Year period. I have mentioned Austria a few times already in this book and I will use this chapter to tie up any remaining loose ends.

It was just my parents and I that set out on this holiday. We arranged to meet at Coventry Airport. Jules was dropping me off and my parents were travelling from Nottingham.

It was a dark, dank December morning when Jules and I arrived. There was no trace of my parents, despite them having set off unusually early as my father had accidentally set the alarm an hour to soon. Now if you know Coventry Airport, you will know it is very difficult to lose someone there. It is little more than a shed, with one other building used for business facilities that doubles as a cafe.

My parents eventually turned up, having been sat in the car for hours. Not only did they set the alarm too early, they also did not realise the café (disguised as a business facility), existed. Having finally made our rendezvous, we said our goodbyes to Jules and went to departures (a separate section of the shed).

The plane took off on schedule and we relaxed for our flight. About an hour and a quarter into the flight, the captain made an announcement; I cannot remember the exact words, but they went something like this:

David Stocks

'Do not be alarmed, but due to technical problems with the navigational system, we have to turn back. Please be aware that the backup navigational systems are working, but the aircraft has to return to Coventry for essential maintenance. On return, a separate plane will be allocated to you and a new flight made as soon as possible.'

Now I have flown on a great deal of flights over the years and this is the first time I have ever had to return to the airport. To everyone's credit, all the passengers remained calm and in good spirits. I wondered what the navigational problem could be. Had the captain lost his glasses and reverted to the backup system (borrowed someone else's glasses?) I somehow believed it couldn't be any more technical than that, a belief conjured up in my mind by the quaintness of Coventry airport.

So, with just half an hour left of the flight remaining, we got stuck on the Coventry aviation ring road and turned back towards Coventry. Just over two hours after leaving Coventry, the captain announced that we had now landed safely back at Coventry.

I was beginning to think it was all a publicity stunt and was secretly being organised by the Coventry tourist board and airport. I rang Jules to let her know that we had arrived safely. She was delighted to hear it and asked what the weather was like. I told her it was much the same as when we had set off and the weather forecast for Coventry that day said the rain would increase as the day went on. Poor Jules, who had returned to

The Celtic Holy Grail Quest

bed after dropping me off at Coventry, thought I was talking gobbledygook. I eventually explained to her that the plane had to return to Coventry, due to navigational problems.

The staff at Coventry pulled out all the stops and soon had us transferred to another flight. This plane included navigational equipment as part of its specification and flew us to Salzburg with no more unscheduled events. Because it was an early flight, we arrived at Salzburg from Coventry, via Coventry, by midday. At which time I phoned Jules to let her know that it was a lovely sunny day in Salzburg.

When you venture into the mountains in Austria you travel back in time, for much of the mountains remain untouched by the so called hand of progress. To me, there is real character locked away in isolated mountain huts. On the Planai, the mountain above Schladming, there is a hut called 'Uncle Willy's Hutte.' Uncle Willy is a woodcarver and every inch of his hut is festooned with woodcarvings. Above his hut is a trail that goes off into the woods. Along this trail, dead trees are transformed into mythical creatures, gnarled faces peering through the branches. Could one such trail lead to the grail? I have ventured long into the woods, but wherever these creatures have led me, their destination has always alluded me.

These huts appear out of the mists, like a winter oasis on dunes of snow. Many a time I have visited a hut by sleigh, drawn as if by magic to their doorsteps. But when trying to retrace the way back by car and foot, the hut can no longer be found. I remember one such mountain hut; it was somewhere on the Ramsau plateau, on the opposite side of the valley to the Planai. We stumbled upon the hut by chance and found ourselves in a dream-world, peopled by grizzled lederhosen clad mountaineers. The hut's owner was 'Eric the Viking.' At least that was what we nicknamed him, after the Viking Warrior of Monty Python fame. He wore a Viking helmet, lederhosen, flippers, goggles and a spear-gun. He also carried a giant horn, which he sounded and proceeded to perform a war dance. A more surreal scene I have not seen before or since. Schnapps was free flowing and we partied into the night. We have tried on many occasions to find this place since, but never has it reappeared. It is a place I now only visit in my dreams, but for just one night I was there and all reality was temporarily suspended.

Who was to say the Fisher King's castle was medieval? All is not always what it appears and maybe the Fisher King takes on many guises. I like to think that in that mountain hut I travelled to the otherworld and who knows, Eric the Viking could have been the Fisher King and his giant horn the Grail? Just maybe? Now what was I supposed to ask the Fisher King?

The Celtic Holy Grail Quest

Chapter 48 Something fishy going on in Stonnall

As mentioned earlier, Jules has a pond containing Koi carp, which she inherited from the previous owner. Koi are a much sought after variety of fish from Asia and have graced many imperial pools. There are many legends associating Koi carp with dragons. One Chinese myth is associated with Dragon Gate falls at Kinkakuji Temple. The legend says that if a carp successfully climbs to the top of the falls, it is magically transformed into a dragon. Only one in ten thousand carp are able to achieve this. In Celtic mythology, water dragons are said to guard the gates to the underworld at sources of water such as springs and wells. You can find the underworld by passing one of these watery guardians. The Loch Ness monster is the most famous water dragon, but they exist all over the British Isles. I cannot see our modern pond being such a gate, but Koi carp are said to bring luck and may help me on my quest.
The nearest thing we had to a dragon was an unusually large Koi carp, nick named Kevin. Jules had built up a good relationship with all the carp, but particularly with the giant Kevin. After renting for some time, Jules eventually purchased the house but the Koi carp were bought as a separate item at quite some expense. This didn't bother Jules, as she was very fond of the fish by then.

A later addition to the household were the cats, who moved in around the same time as me,

David Stocks

October 2006. Now I have previously introduced you to the cats and in particular their extrovert personalities. One tale I have not yet told is Tilly's introduction to the pond. Now Tilly is a very curious cat and when she arrived at Jules' house, she went out exploring and soon found the pond. Not content to wander around the pond, Tilly had to jump up onto the wall that makes up the edge of the pond and take a precarious route that zigzagged between the main pond and the drainage pool. Perhaps she was searching for a dragon? It was while she was wending her way across this, staring at the fish, that she lost her balance and her little kitten-cat paws wavered for one heart stopping moment in the air, before the laws of gravity took over and she dropped unceremoniously water-wards. The look of horror on her face as she gave in to her fate was heart rending. Unfortunately for Tilly she didn't fall in the nice clean pond among the fish, she dropped into the green slime of the drainage pool and disappeared with a squelch. The time in the slime was a matter of milliseconds; not wanting to stay within the soggy embrace of green algae for a moment longer than required, Tilly propelled herself back out of the pool. What entered the pond as a dainty, clean, but overly curious grey and white cat, exited the pool as a jet propelled, howling, fluorescent green swamp monster. There was no consoling Tilly-cat, her pride had been mortally wounded. She took her dignity, slime and all, back into the house. Jules pursued this howling swamp-thing through every room, where

The Celtic Holy Grail Quest

she proceeded to trail green slime behind her all over the carpets and furniture. Jules eventually cornered the creature from the swamps and wrapped the wailing, biting, clawing creature in a towel. What emerged from the towel some minutes later was a very sorrowful, ruffled, sulky, but clean grey and white Tilly-cat. There have been no more swamp monster incidents since.

We realised the full purpose of the drainage pool some months later, when the water level had reduced to a minimum and algae started to collect on the pond. We called upon the expertise of Paul (the original owner of the house and pond), to help us unblock the drainage. This Paul did with some efficiency as he had originally designed the pond and owns a fishery. Taking careful note of everything he did, we thanked Paul for his help and thought that was the end of it. We didn't find a dragon hiding in the murky depths; the nearest we ever came to seeing a dragon was when Tilly transformed into a howling swamp-monster. Later that day, I was sat in the office upstairs in the front of the house, when a net appeared underneath the window. 'Hmmn,' I thought ... 'fishing net,' I thought. The net bobbed up and down a bit ... 'strange,' I thought. Then the doorbell rang. I stood up and looked down, only to discover that the net was on a long pole, the other end of which was being held by the man now ringing our doorbell. He was about five feet ten in height with grey hair and was dressed casually. A close fitting woollen hat was pulled down over his

David Stocks

head. The one outstanding feature I remember about him was that he was wearing thick, deep, brick red rubber gloves, of the kind road workers wear. 'Strange,' I thought. Jules came running upstairs and muttered something about him being a weirdo with a penchant for her fish and she asked me to see him off. Before I managed to get up and go downstairs to greet our friend with the rubber gloves and fish net, our unexpected visitor departed. We watched him leave and I wondered after he left where his net had gone, as he appeared to be no longer carrying it. He turned into a driveway a few houses down and I assumed that he must have already put the net down at his house and that he was a neighbour - albeit a somewhat unusual neighbour.

I thought nothing of it for the rest of the day and it wasn't until we were sitting outside later, enjoying a beer in the early spring sunshine, that Jules mentioned him again. Well not so much him, more the net. Apparently when she had been taking the rubbish out, she went down the side of the house and found the mysterious fishing net lying on the floor. It had either been thrown over the gate or pushed under it. The mystery began to deepen. We now knew why the unexpected visitor didn't have a net when he turned into his driveway. It was hidden down the side of our house. I enquired about the circumstances of Jules' previous encounter with our eccentric visitor. Jules explained that she had met him once before, while walking up the gully that ran past her house. It

The Celtic Holy Grail Quest

was about a year ago and he asked her whether she still had the fish in the back pond. She said she had and he told her that he would be round for some later as it was healthy for the fish to take them out of the water on occasions. Jules, with raised eyebrows, confidently told him that the fish belonged to her and *she* would decide what was good for them. He then proceeded to tell Jules that the previous owner, Paul, had told him that he could help himself to some. He appeared later that day in the same heavy duty rubber gloves and with the same fishing net, instructing Jules that he would show her how to take the fish out of the pond. Jules told him in no uncertain terms that she was not going to go along with this instruction and he went away. She hadn't seen him since until this latest encounter. She had phoned Paul at the time and he had said that he knew nothing of him.

We decided to give Paul another call in case he had seen anything 'fishy' going on when he had called round earlier that day. Paul again said that he knew nothing of this man, but that a large net had gone missing when he had lived there. It was one that he had brought back from his fishery and seemed to fit the description of our man's net very well. He advised us to call the police.

We called the police and related the strange events of the pond full of valuable Koi carp, a ten foot fishing net and a fifty-or-so year old man wearing heavy duty gloves and a Benny hat. The policeman on the other end of the line did well to keep the humour out of his voice and recorded the details diligently.

Now we had begun to formulate ideas about our unexpected visitor. Paul is a nice guy, but he is not quiet about letting it be known the value of things, such as Koi carp. We decided the mysterious man could well be a burglar, looking to pinch some of the Koi carp, with the thought of making a quick buck. He had been round earlier that day and finding no one in, had taken the opportunity to slide the ten foot fishing net under the gate. He had probably pushed it down the shady side of the house with the intention of returning later to avail himself of some of the pond's contents. The more we thought about this, the more certain we were that this was his plan.

We were by now convinced by our theory, so late that night we set a trap. We left the net exactly where it was, so that he wouldn't suspect anything and went to bed. Before settling down, we opened the windows so that we would hear him if he 'scaled' the fence and left our jeans at the bottom of the bed ready to hop into. We also had our digital camera to hand so that we could take a picture of him in the act. All was set; that night we would 'net' us a thief, the international fish thief, 'Slippery Fin.'

To our dismay, however, despite one false alarm when we thought we heard something, nothing happened. It was a big 'net down.'

The Celtic Holy Grail Quest

We visited some friends the next day near Stratford and after a very enjoyable time we returned home to find a policeman waiting for us on our arrival. We invited him into our home and recounted our fishy tail of nets, rubber gauntlets and slippery characters. He wondered where exactly the would-be thief was planning on keeping the fish, at which point I told him about the dream I had the night before. In the dream the thief had 'scaled' the fence, acquired the net and hooked out our prize fish, returning home with his catch. He had then sent us a ransom note, made from cut up newspaper letters, demanding a large sum of money for the safety of the fish. At the bottom of the note was a picture of Kevin in a bathtub. The poor policeman recorded all the details meticulously, handed us his card and said if we spotted anything 'fishy' going on again, to let him know. With this he left the house somewhat bemused by the whole incident.

The carp have brought us much pleasure and I firmly believe they have brought me luck on the quest for the Grail.
They are very good for stress relief and nothing can be more pleasurable and therapeutic than sitting at the edge of the pond watching them swim on a summer's day. They form a most beautiful myriad of bright colours swirling through the water, causing an occasional loud splash when one jumps across the water.

David Stocks

Chapter 49 The structure of the universe and interconnectedness

During my search for the Grail, I have trawled library archives, queried databases, visited far flung places, talked to amazing people, read numerous books and travelled the information highways of the Internet. I have amalgamated a mind boggling array of information, which I have formulated into solid ideas, concepts and theories. From these postulations I am going to question the very nature of reality and with that knowledge undergo a final test and the realisation of the Grail quest.
So what is reality? Let us first take a look at the structure of the universe. I am not a theoretical physicist, astronomer or scientist of any kind. I therefore lay out my arguments in layman's terms, for as a layman this is all I can do. I leave the complex science and mathematics to those better qualified to do so. It is not the actual science I am trying to portray, it is the underlying ideas. Forgive me for any misconceptions that I may have. I openly invite debate, for without argument we would be stuck with limited viewpoints.
Having recently read an article suggesting that the universe is not expanding randomly - which would have the mass more or less spread uniformly throughout the universe - but rather in fractal patterns increasing in size the further out you look into the universe, I decided to look deeper into fractals. Fractals are found everywhere,

The Celtic Holy Grail Quest

particularly in nature. They are repeating patterns that are complete copies of larger or smaller patterns in a particular subject. For example, a fern has a distinctive pattern, but if you look at the tips of fern leaves you will find the very same pattern repeated on a smaller scale. Similar fractals occur in snowflakes, flowers, tree bark etc. Comparisons can be drawn between nature's examples and the universe, which has fractal patterns of stars that repeat in the star patterns of galaxies, then galaxy clusters and ever on outwards.

One of the problems with a fractal universe is the fact that we only see fractals in luminous matter, which makes up just fifteen per cent of the universe. The remaining eighty five per cent is made up of dark matter, which is invisible. A recent study looking at the gravitational effects of dark matter on the stars has shown spiral fractal patterns in the dark matter too. The densest regions of dark matter correspond to the densest regions of luminous matter, with vast empty voids in between.

Each individual fractal contains an exact copy of the next larger fractal and so on, in much the same way holograms work. A hologram is a three dimensional photograph created by shining a laser beam onto an object and then bouncing a second laser beam off the light reflected by the first. This creates an interference pattern which is recorded on photographic film. What is most interesting

David Stocks

about holograms is that when they are cut up, each and every piece of the hologram contains the entire image in exact detail, but on a smaller scale. Similar replications in fractals suggest that any given point in the universe contains a smaller copy of the entire universe.

However, I hear you say, 'If the big bang explodes chaotically, then how do fractal patterns emerge?' The answer to that question is to look into whether chaos is in fact totally random.

Edward Lorenz, a meteorologist, looked into the patterns of weather that would emerge if the current weather of two nearby starting points was studied. The plotted trajectories frequently ended up in different lobes, which corresponded to calm or stormy weather. This takes the form of a butterfly shape and gave rise to the 'Butterfly Effect' metaphor:

'The flapping of a butterfly's wings in China today may cause a tornado in Kansas tomorrow.'

See Diagram below for example image of the butterfly effect.

The Celtic Holy Grail Quest

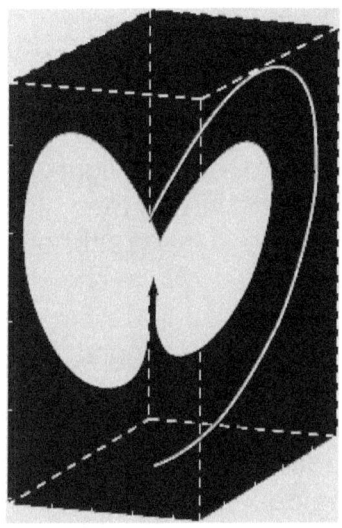

This is just one example of how out of chaos and complexity, fractal patterns emerge. Numerous studies show that supposedly chaotic systems form non random deterministic outcomes.

Under certain conditions chaos is not random.

British chemist, James E. Lovelock, and the American biologist, Lynn Margulis, came up with the 'Gaia Hypothesis' of complementary evolution of life and environment, named after Gaia, the ancient Greek goddess of the earth.

This echoes the Celtic way of life, of living in harmony with Mother Earth and their gods.

James Lovelock explains it as, 'The earth's living matter, air, oceans, and land surface form a complex system which can be seen as a single organism and which has the capacity to keep our planet a fit place for life.'

What if this self regulating system extends right out into the universe, with the structure of the universe maintained by a balance in the matter of stars, pulsars and black holes?

The model of the universe is self replicating as I see it. British Physicist, Ernest Rutherford, postulated that the atom resembled a miniature solar system, with light, negatively charged electrons orbiting around the dense, positively charged nucleus, just as the planets orbit around the sun.

Looking at the non-chaotic structure of the universe, starting with subatomic particles, plants, oceans, the weather, stars, galaxies and outwards; these all display fractal patterns and there appears to be an inherent design built in to the very fabric of the universe.

The underlying structure of the universe appears to follow a fractal design.

To back this idea up, a French Astrophysicist, Laurent Nottale, has set out to extend Einstein's principle of relativity, in which the laws of physics remain the same regardless of the motion of the observer - to a theory in which the laws of physics would remain the same regardless of the scale at

The Celtic Holy Grail Quest

which the universe is being observed.

Guess what the conclusions were? That the underlying space-time of such a theory would have to be fractal.

Now we have seen the self replicating nature of fractals extending out into the universe, I am going to take a look at dimensionless points, as proposed by Swedish polymath Swedenborg, in his book 'The Principia.'

Dimensionless points have no extension in space. Not being restricted to one location, they are universally present, existing everywhere. Because the points are the connecting point to the infinite, they have infinite energy. Every infinitesimal dimensionless point contains an entire copy of the universe, much the same as a hologram or a fractal. Swedenborg also predicted the spiralling of particles as a constraint of the dimensionless points moving away from the infinite over time and ultimately the spiralling of galaxies, such as the Milky Way.

Dimensionless points mirror a view that I have had for a long time that everything is connected.

This in turn mirrors Celtic beliefs, with seers or 'fey' people who have the gift of far sight. They had a world-view in which everything is connected; the boundaries between one person and another, past and future, appeared to melt.

David Stocks

The interconnectedness of everything is a strong theme that has run throughout this quest. It is this very feature present in everything, that ultimately leads me to my goal, that of the Grail.

The Celtic Holy Grail Quest

Chapter 50 Angelic light and dark matter

As we have seen we are in a universe that is largely made up of undetected dark matter. I am now going to move on to a hypothetical theory on angels. Everything I have read, seen and experienced over the past few years has led me to believe in the existence of angels.

Firstly I am going to theorise that dark matter is negative energy (negative emotions) and that luminous matter is positive energy (positive emotions). This doesn't mean that dark matter is evil, it just casts a shadow over you, and it has a negative pull on your psyche. All this negative energy causes a lot of people to look deep inside them. If you can keep afloat and not drown in the pit of sorrow, this can be very beneficial, for with introspection comes creativity. A lot of famous artists, writers and poets are naturally depressive people, but these people have produced some of the greatest creative works in the world. I encourage anyone suffering from depression to engage their mind in something, be creative and laugh in the face of adversity.

I propose that man's inherent instinct to look at the negative side of things and particularly to remember the bad things that have happened, rather than the good things, is not only due to evolutionary forces where man needed to remember what is dangerous to survive, but in the

David Stocks

ability for man to sense dark matter. Note: this is only a conjecture and a very radical conjecture at that, with no evidence to back it up. If this is the case however, it would explain negative people, of which there are a lot, as being receptors for dark matter. Most people readily pick up luminous matter as well, although not in great quantities. It counteracts the dark matter and balances out their personalities. Depressed people pick up hardly any luminous matter, but are sole receptors for dark matter, hence their dark, moody personalities.

So where do angels fit into this? I believe everyone is an angel in essence, with their physical bodies being their earthly form. I believe everyone has a soul mate. People who receive luminous matter are attracted to people who receive dark matter.

In effect, angels of light find their soul mate in dark angels. Jules came to me in a dream as an angel of light and she has found a soul mate in me, a dark angel. The notion of opposites attract applies. The distinction becomes less obvious the more balance of luminous and dark matter reception there is in each individual. A very romantic notion, I know, but one that I am fond of. I feel a Bohemian side in me, when I think of harmony between light and dark angels.

>   From tortured wastelands of the soul,
>   To fertile astral plains,

The Celtic Holy Grail Quest

I sit beside my angel,
And drink from the pool of love.

So how do angels appear in another realm? Accounts of people who claim to have visited angels, including Swedenborg, state that it is very hard to express angels in words, particularly angelic speech. Angelic speech expresses such a staggering array of concepts, messages and meanings, that it is impossible to record them in words.

Spiritualism and quests in the Celtic tradition are closely linked to poetry. My quest for the Holy Grail is a very spiritual journey. Poetry may be a way of portraying angelic speech to the best of our abilities, as many poems form ideas with numerous interpretations and messages from a minimum of words.

Angelic words at once display the infinitesimal side of reality. Yet because everything is linked, it is impossible to think of one thing without linking it to everything else. The core principle is that of unity. The Celtic Bards were master wordsmiths, their words connecting them to the spirit world. It is through regaining the mastery of words of the Celtic Bard or seer, that I can make the connection to the otherworld and locate the Grail.

From a sacred grove I beg a gift,
On the eve of Yule during the darkest hour.
From the venerable yew with grace I make,

David Stocks

A bow of wood sprung from death's own marrow.

With a string spun from finest flax,
I notch a heartwood arrow.
And draw the bow against the silvery moon,
Arching along its crescent silhouette.

Water flows like quicksilver,
From the caverns of the underworld.
I take sight across this brook,
As another year turns over.

I let fly the arrow like a star burning bright,
Piercing death's domain.
With its flight my soul does pass,
To where my ancestors do dwell.

I step where I should not tread,
Pierced by the kiss of an arrow.
There I lay my demons to rest,
On death's hallowed ground.

I lay in a stream of sacred salmon,
Awash with hidden knowledge.
And emerge reborn in a shaft of light,
At the start of the year and a bright new life.

The Celtic Holy Grail Quest

Chapter 51 Desperate times

In the last six months my life had radically changed. I had come off medication in one fell swoop and awoken from a dream-like trance. Functioning again, I felt the need to prove myself in the real world. Having had my confidence knocked in the library at which I was working, I decided to put all my efforts into a new future. I moved in with Jules and we decided to start a business together. I won't go into the details of our business venture, for that is a story unto itself, but I will mention the impact it had on our lives.

Jules was struggling to support the both of us on one salary and having had a good idea for a business enterprise, she left her job and we committed ourselves fully to the business. Now whatever I say next, this business venture is the best thing I ever did. We worked night and day, seven days a week to put together the business. From a proposal, detailed business plan to premises at a brilliant location, we learnt a great deal over a period of a few months.

The trouble was we were very low on funds and were struggling from day to day to keep a roof over our heads. Despite having a fantastic business idea that everyone loved and a business plan that impressed, we kept getting knock backs. Coupled with these knock backs was my severe mood swings, when I would go from a normal functioning person, if not a totally happy individual, to an utterly despondent human being in the depths of despair. It ended up with Jules having to keep a constant watch on me, including right throughout the night, to make sure I did myself no harm. We had difficulty in getting help from the local Primary Care Trust, mainly due to the fact that I had suffered from depression for six years now and was classed as incurable, with a mood disorder.

Every time we had a knock back and thought that we had reached an all time low and things could not get any worse, they did. Eventually we found that we just could not sink any lower and we reached an all time rock bottom. We had everything set up for the business, premises, support and belief from some high powered people, all we needed was some funding. We were offered a majority of this by our local bank and as a stop gap we asked them for a temporary overdraft or loan until we had secured all the funding. This was turned down and the next thing we knew, within a gap of about fifteen minutes the business loan offer was rescinded, which we found to be very suspicious. On top of this my mood swings had got worse and worse, with the added factor of anxiety, which caused me to vent uncontrollable outbursts of anger. We could not get help from the local Primary Care Trust, we had absolutely no money in the bank and we had a highly viable business, but with no capital to back it up. That's when we realised we had hit rock

The Celtic Holy Grail Quest

bottom!

It is a strange feeling when you know there is no further down you can go, a kind of acceptance comes upon you, and so we decided to accept that whatever will be, will be. The only way from here was up! As long as we stuck together, nothing and no-one could possibly harm us. We mulled it over and decided that even in the worse case scenario of bankruptcy, we could start again with all the new found skills we had gained from setting up a business. If we lost everything now, we would forge a new bright future for ourselves.

Despite the calm resolution we had made, my anxiety continued to increase and my mood swings became ever more severe. These eventually reached a peak and I had to be admitted to hospital. The Primary Care Trust had finally realised that I needed professional treatment and time out away from the pressures of the real world and close contact with people. Time out for me was by then essential in order to regroup myself, get my head together and prepare myself for getting back in to society and building a fresh new life with Jules. We decided that while I was in hospital, Jules would continue trying to get the business off the ground and if it ultimately failed, we would still keep the idea for future. We were not going to give up on it that easily.

During the course of all these events, the completion of my quest was picking up speed, until the influx of ideas and insights I was receiving was thundering through my mind like a runaway train that I couldn't get off. I was being bombarded with information that was going to help me reach my goal, that of the Holy Grail, and I couldn't get the ideas down fast enough. My notebook was flooding with my hastily jotted notes and it was all I could do to stem the tide and form some concrete conclusions, conclusions that would eventually lead me to the Holy Grail.

What I have written in this book is just the tip of the iceberg, most of which lies deep underwater. I hit on an untapped stream of insights, ideas and concepts that I can't switch off from. I don't know if this is a blessing or a curse.
Hold on tight and join me for the mind opening, dizzying, heart stopping conclusion of this quest.

The Celtic Holy Grail Quest

Chapter 52 Potential, possibilities and precognition

Every decision we make has potential, the universe is full of possibilities, and every action is the realisation of potential. When a baby is born it is a body of pure potential. All the information a baby receives from the outside world through its senses are amalgamated and analysed, and a number of potentials can come out of resulting actions that the baby takes. For example, when a baby sees a teddy bear, there are a number of different potentials: grab it, hug it, crawl away from it or hide (could be a red teddy bear and the baby doesn't like red), kiss it, bite it, or suck it.

At any one moment there are a number of different potentials in the universe. Here is another example: a seed pod falls from a tree. What will happen to that seed pod?

The seed pod could just drop down directly below the tree; the seed pod may or may not germinate and grow into another tree; the seed pod could drift on the wind a short distance or get carried thousands of miles on the wind; the seed pod again may or may not germinate, but it could possibly grow into a tree, thousands of miles away from its parent tree; the seed pod could be picked up by a bird and be used to make a nest; the seed pod could drop to the ground and then later be eaten by an animal. This creature could then travel to another location and digest the seeds, after which the droppings from the animal containing the seed could be exactly the right mixture for fertilisation, and eventually germinate and grow into a tree.

As you can see there is endless potential for any given event. So you may, therefore, think things are just totally random and no event could possibly be mapped out in the future.

There is however strong evidence for precognition, although scientists will argue against it, as you can't reproduce it in a laboratory. The evidence is still there to be looked at though.

Nostradamus is the most famous precognitive; in his book of quatrains (four-line verses) he described major events yet to come. He first rose to fame with a prediction, the 35th quatrain, which spoke of how a 'young lion' would vanquish 'the elder one' in combat, with a blow that would 'pierce the eyes in their golden cage - two wounds in one, thence to meet a cruel death.'

This appears to be an all too accurate account of a jousting competition held in July 1559 (after the quatrain was written), in which King Henry II of France received a blow from his opponent's lance that sent splinters through his visor, piercing his eye and lodging in his brain. Henry died 10 days later.

The Celtic Holy Grail Quest

Now sceptics will argue all sorts of things to make this event not the subject of a prediction, mainly on the grounds of the multitude of different interpretations that can be made of the Nostradamus quatrains. This may be true of a lot of his quatrains, but this one to me seems to be pretty clear cut. No doubt somebody will take great pleasure in refuting this.

Of great interest, the Celts have a long tradition of poet-seers who were able to see signs, and by using their intuition could temporarily part the veil of time.

There are a number of other predictions that I have come across too. Think of it like intuition; have you ever thought that the phone is going to ring and almost immediately afterwards the phone has rung? Or have you been going to ring someone and then the next moment that person has called you? Or perhaps you have even thought about someone that you have not seen for a long time and then they get in touch with you, or you meet them in a chance encounter? I am sure everyone has at least once in their lives had some kind of premonition. A sceptic of course would just put these events down to coincidence. This is a topic I will move onto after this. A lot of prophecies come to us in dreams.

Here are some prophetic examples: -

Soccer fan Adrian Hayward won £25,000 after

David Stocks

dreaming that Liverpool's Xabi Alonso scored a goal from his own half. Hayward placed a £200 bet at the odds of 125-1 that Alonso would score from his own half at some point in the season. On 7th January, the dream came true when the Spaniard scored against Luton Town in the FA Cup third round. (Source: Fortean Times, February 2007).

John Godfrey, Lord Kilbracken, who died in the summer of 2006:-
In 1946, while an undergraduate at Oxford, he dreamt the winners of two horse races. He backed them and they won. There were eight further winning dreams, the last two of which he recorded, dated, deposited in the safe of the Oxford postmaster and reported in the Daily Mirror. The horses won, the Mirror verified the contents of the safe and offered Godfrey a job as a racing tipster. Thereafter the dreams ceased, until they returned briefly to give him the winner of the 1958 Grand National. (Source: Fortean Times, January 2007).

Alain van Dael, 36, dreamed he won the Belgian Lotto with the numbers 2, 6, 9, 11, 40, 41. Then he did - and on the 13th of October 2006 he collected £270,000 in Antwerp. (Source: Fortean Times, February 2007, original source: Sun newspaper, 14th October 2006).

A great Buddhist master of the 8th century, Padmasambhava, predicted that the Dhama

The Celtic Holy Grail Quest

would spread in the west 'when the iron bird flies and horses run on wheels.' (Source: Practical meditation with Buddhist principles, Hinkler Books Pty Ltd, 2006).

As you can see there are a number of prophecies that have come true. I would now like to move on to the subject of coincidences. I am constantly having coincidences occur around me, as I am sure many other people do. The amount of coincidences and the nature of some of these coincidences appear to me to be too extreme, to lie within the realms of probability. Note: these are just a few coincidences that I have had, there are many more.

Examples:

I went to see some drag racing at Santa Pod race track with my brother-in-law and a friend of his. We discussed how we were going to get there before the day and decided to go in his friend's car who I had never met. We decided not to travel in mine as it was new and had a very sensitive alarm i.e. the alarm was liable to go off with the vibrations of the jet engines in some of the dragsters. When his friend arrived, he was driving my old car that I had part exchanged at a garage recently. I repeat I had never met him; he came from a different part of Nottingham and I had sold the car in a part exchange deal to a garage.

Another incident occurred while I was working in a

coffee shop in Nottingham. A customer came in and commented that he was pleased that he could get a coffee while in the town, as although there was a nice coffee shop in the village where he lived, it didn't open very early. I asked him what village he was from and he told me, 'Radcliffe.' Somewhat surprised I replied that I had just moved there. He then went on to ask me whereabouts in Radcliffe I lived. I told him, 'Lorne Grove.' This surprised him and he said that he used to live in Lorne Grove. I then ventured to ask him which house he had lived in. He told me that he had lived in a flat at number twelve. Even more startled, I somewhat tentatively asked him whether it was the top flat that he had lived in. The answer was, 'Yes' - the very flat that I had just moved into!

In yet another incident, I was setting up a new bank account. I filled in all the forms and handed them in. I got a phone call later that week from the bank asking if I could call in, as they needed another signature. I went into the bank during the course of the next week and was just in the process of asking one of the bank's employees about my new account, when I got a phone call on my mobile. I apologised and took the call. It was a lady from the bank calling. She apologised for calling me at work, but she needed me to come in to sign a form and could I make it soon. I was somewhat taken aback. I told her I was in the bank at this moment and was just in the process of asking about the form. She paused, and then asked, 'Are you the gentleman in the white shirt?'

The Celtic Holy Grail Quest

You can guess what my response was!

I was playing a CD one evening, a Turin Brakes track, and Jules commented that it reminded her of when she last knew me. This was six years previous when I had my first breakdown. She said the track was on a compilation CD that was out at the time. She went and got the CD and read the date on the back of it, which was 16th April 2001. This was the first time she had looked at it in years and the current date was 16th April 2007, exactly six years ago to the day.

So, I have written about precognition and coincidence, but what else is there? What about telepathy? I will give just one example of this - but there are many more – by recounting one of the many psychic incidents that Swedenborg experienced.

Swedenborg, who I have previously mentioned, was at dinner in Gothenberg, when he suddenly got up and left the party looking pale and shaken. When asked what was wrong, he replied that a fire had just broken out in Stockholm, some 300 miles away. The fire had started in Sodermalm where his house was and was spreading quickly. Restless, Swedenborg soon announced that a friend's house was now in ruins. He continued to be agitated until about eight o'clock - two hours after he had originally announced it - when he told the party, with relief, that the fire had now been extinguished. That evening, the Governor was told of Swedenborg's vision. The next day Swedenborg retold him the events in Stockholm the previous night in minute detail. Swedenborg had his vision on a Saturday and on the following Monday a messenger arrived at Gothenburg describing the fire exactly as Swedenborg had described it, with all the timings and events surrounding it being the same.

From this evidence the following conclusions can be drawn:-

Everything is connected; there is more than just coincidence at work. If we use Swedenborg's dimensionless points, every point contains everything within the universe, including time. This means everything is connected to everything else by any one event in the universe; no matter what its location is in space and time it can be accessed from any other location in space and time. I believe that every event sends a ripple effect out into the space-time fabric of the universe.

Therefore, if this is the case, then everything is preordained, even though you make choices, those choices are preordained. You may think that having read this text that you are going to make changes in your life and I say, 'Do so, if those changes are going to have a positive beneficial effect for you.' Those choices may have been preordained, but to you they are still choices. The fact that you are reading this is preordained, but that has not stopped you making the choices to get to this juncture. Without a genuine seer - and be warned there are a great many charlatans -

The Celtic Holy Grail Quest

you will be unable to see what choices you make in the future. Therefore to you, you are still exhibiting free will. Whatever course you take is supported by universal forces, which are preordained. Fate is mapped out for you and therefore you have nothing to fear.

David Stocks

Chapter 53 Companionship, sorrow, metamorphosis and revelation

I end my quest where I began; like a Celtic labyrinth I have followed the twists and turns of life's maze, back and forth, meeting all the challenges on the way in my quest for the Celtic Holy Grail. I find myself back at the beginning of the labyrinth, back in hospital, suffering from severe depression. But it is a much changed person that stands here than at the beginning and it is with a lot greater understanding of life's mysteries that I return here. It is here in the Dorothy Pattison hospital in Walsall that I near the end of my quest and grasp the meaning of the Celtic Holy Grail.

I have come to a number of conclusions during the course of my Grail quest. They have given me many insights to the origins of the universe and life, but I have still got to achieve my quest and ask the question 'Whom does the Grail serve?'

Before I dare pose that question, I need to examine the thought processes that have brought me to this juncture on this quest and the surrounding circumstances.

It was the night of Wednesday 14th March 2007 that I arrived in the ward at the Dorothy Pattison hospital. I was immediately greeted by my fellows, for want of a better word, inmates. Now I am not

The Celtic Holy Grail Quest

saying inmates in the sense that it was like a prison, as it was far from it. The staff and nurses were there to care for us and help us to recuperate. To this end they couldn't have been nicer. I am saying inmates, because for our own safety, we were under constant surveillance and were restricted on times we could leave the ward. The guys that greeted me were the friendliest bunch of people you could possibly hope to meet. They welcomed me like a long lost friend, pulled up a chair for me and made me a cup of tea. I felt an immediate empathy with them and knew that I had come to the right place. I could feel the tension draining from me immediately.

Over the next few days I got to know my fellow inmates a lot better and I found friends in all of them. There were two people in particular that I got on with most: Jeff, who was ever so much a gentlemen, and Ian, who was a lot younger than me, but with whom I hit it off straight away. I could see in him much of what I had been suffering and we shared the same tastes in Alternative Rock and Heavy Metal music. What's more, he had the voice of a rock star; I particularly likened him to Kurt Cobain and that is high praise indeed.

It was with this comforting feeling of companionship that the tension began to ooze out of me and I spent a lot of time reading various texts that gave me insight and inspiration. This helped me to come within reach of my ultimate goal, that of the Celtic Holy Grail. While I was

David Stocks

reading, I was constantly making notes as ideas and inspiration came upon me. When I finally had time to reflect, I realised what a productive time it was. I took to revamping my book, distilling the contents and creating a new more contiguous text, structuring it in such a way that it at once became more accessible and enjoyable to read. I listened to music all the time I was doing this and I found this both relaxing and stimulating at the same time. Music is the catalyst of the mind, the source of inspiration, the bringer of intuition.

And so we approach the end of my quest, the time of conclusions, a time of introspection, analysis and, finally, revelation. Let me warn you who have journeyed with me thus far, it is not all positive and light, in fact far from it. I have had to journey down many dark corridors to get here. This day in particular has been dark and I would not recommend that anyone goes there, but out of the ashes of this day, a spark of hope has enlightened my soul and the Celtic Holy Grail is almost within my grasp.

This day is March 18th 2007, Mothering Sunday.

It is with some trepidation that I approach this keyboard and recount the events of this day. I type on, not in the desire to finish the book, but in the

The Celtic Holy Grail Quest

desire to relate the events of the day while its effects are still coursing through me. I need to paint in words to depict a truer picture of my feelings at this time, to vent the intensity of my emotions and to portray the full meaning of what I have found.

I woke up some time before 6 am this morning. I could not sleep anymore as my mind was racing. I put on my headphones and listened to some music. It was a Pink Floyd album. I started reading one of my books, a particularly interesting book about a Swedish Polymath (someone who has proficient skills and understanding of many different subjects) called Swedenborg, who I have mentioned previously. It is written by Gary Lachman, a former rock musician and songwriter. I was introduced to it by an article he had written in the magazine, the Fortean Times. The book is called 'Into the interior: discovering Swedenborg.' It is about Swedenborg's quest into his inner self, to understand the meaning of dreams and visions he had been having, to decode and present the true meaning of the Bible scriptures to the rest of the world. It was a book that I could relate to, as I have had many dreams, visions and unexplained voices that I was trying to make sense of. Reading this book has given me many insights into my mind and how the mind works, and ultimately the nature of reality. These insights I have been noting down in a notebook, as they come upon me.

David Stocks

Another book that has also been a great influence on me that I have already mentioned in a previous chapter is 'The book of secrets,' by Deepak Chopra. Again it has inspired many insights; it is a very spiritual book, with key clues to the nature of existence. Both Depak Chopra and Swedenborg have scientific backgrounds, but are very spiritual too. This has given them a broad outlook that has helped them reach some startling conclusions. As with Swedenborg's book I have noted down any thoughts and inspirations that have been awoken in me while reading the book. In the past few weeks I have been reaching for my notebook on countless occasions, as I have begun to build up a picture of reality and all that it entails. My findings I have noted down in the preceding chapters - with an ultimate revelation based on information I have gained from these books and many magazine articles, both scientific and esoterically - to be revealed here.

What I am about to divulge is my own personal views on creation, reality and the meaning of life. I am comfortable with these for my own personal perspective on things, but readily admit I am no expert in spirituality, science or philosophy, but rather more consider me a student polymath. For this reason, I ask my fellow journeymen to reach their own conclusions and search inside themselves for the truth. I hope what I reveal here will help others on their quest. One thing I have learned on this quest is to think outside of the box. Look at all the available data from as many

The Celtic Holy Grail Quest

different sources as possible and look at it from a new angle, don't follow any pre-conceived ideas. Don't follow a straight line of linear thinking, but think sideways.

Returning to the main focus of today's events; while I was reading the book, I heard the lyrics from one verse of a Pink Floyd song called 'Money.' They happened to coincide with what I had been thinking and saying to people over the past few weeks, that money is evil. The lyrics are, 'Money is the root of all evil.' Never a truer word spoken. When you analyse it, what happens when money becomes involved? Drugs are sold and people are enslaved to prostitution, for the sake of money. Wars break out, because countries desire the riches to be found in other countries - this could be because the country has rich resources in oil, for instance. Family's break up over arguments about money, be it inheritance or gifts. If mankind was not greedy and shared money and resources, there would be more than enough for everyone.

I will now return to the topic of coincidence. I feel there is a lot more going on than coincidence. Scientists will say that there is always an explanation for coincidence, but my feelings are that everything is interconnected. I see coincidences as hidden signposts in life, hints that there is more to be explored within the universe than what is understood at the moment.

David Stocks

The next event describes my experience of revelation. Before I describe it, I want to take you back to the Arthurian legend of the Holy Grail. Of all the mighty knights that started the quest it was the humble Perceval, who had been brought up by his widowed mother in the forest and had never seen a knight, a sword, or a horse, who eventually found the grail. A key point to note in this is that the name Perceval literally translates to 'pierce-the-veil.' Following his spirit journey I eventually managed to pierce the veil of reality.

Still listening to Pink Floyd I then had my moment of inspiration and revelation. One of the reasons that I play music is to drown out the voices that I hear, as described in previous chapters. The fact that I can hear voices and the voices appear real to me means that I have generated that reality. If my mind has generated that reality it therefore stands to reason that it has also generated what we class as reality and that the whole of reality is a construct of our minds.

If you find this hard to grasp, think about when you have woken from a dream, a dream that has been so vivid that everything in it has seemed real. All the senses have been engaged: Touch, sight, sound, smell and hearing. You have woken up from it convinced that everything in the dream is real and it has taken a while for you to realise that you have been dreaming. That dream to you at the time was real, but it was all in fact constructed

The Celtic Holy Grail Quest

in the mind, so if the mind can construct reality in a dream, then why can't it construct reality itself?

Within our minds is the spark of creation from which all else springs, the physical world and the physical body; we are all created from this spark. If you look inside your physical body and follow the labyrinth of undulating matter that makes up the brain and search deep enough, etched on the surface of the brain is a label 'made in the mind.' Everything we perceive is a construct of the mind.

Throughout this journey as a Celtic warrior in search of the Holy Grail, I have been aware of the butterfly as a symbol that keeps cropping up. I see this as a sign from the creator, be it the essence of my mind or some mighty creator (note there is a lot of evidence for intelligent design.) 'The Book of Secrets' by Deepak Chopra tells you to look for signs. This I have done and I have seen many signs throughout this book, but the main one being the butterfly.

The final lesson that I can learn from the butterfly is that of transformation. I started this quest as a caterpillar, blind to the insights that I needed to transform me. Throughout the journey I gained these insights and then I went back to basics, nutrients within my mother's womb, waiting to form into a baby. As a caterpillar entered a cocoon, I entered the womb, these nutrients combined and the caterpillar (I) was reborn as a butterfly.

David Stocks

In many beliefs a baby is born knowing everything and gradually forgets it through life. The truth is that everything is nothing, a baby is an empty receptacle waiting to take on data through all its senses, and with that data build a picture of reality. This pure state of nothingness is the essence of being and a baby is in fact born with the seed of potential to nurture into whatever reality it likes. That seed can be compared to Swedenborg's dimensionless points connected to everything else, with infinite energy and infinite potential for creation.

I continue now with trepidation as I take you up to this present moment and recount the rest of the day's events.

As I type this, there is a policeman stationed outside the room next door. The reason he is there is as follows:

At about 9:55 am this morning I got a knock at the door; this was immediately after I had finally reached my ultimate conclusions on the mechanisms of reality, the understandings that were bringing the Grail within my grasp. I felt satisfied; a burden had been lifted off my shoulders and I no longer had to seek any more answers as all the answers I needed were there. But I still had one final lesson to learn and this was my biggest lesson of all.

One of the nurses entered my room and said

The Celtic Holy Grail Quest

something to me. I didn't hear what he said, as I was listening to my music at the time, but I acknowledged him anyway. He disappeared and I tried to regain my concentration, as I made my final few notes. I then glanced at my watch and it was nearly ten o'clock. I realised the nurse must have been telling me my visitors had arrived and that I now must be keeping them waiting. Visiting times were 10:00 am to 12:00 midday and my family visited me at ten every morning.

The next events unfolded. I stepped out of the room and the nurse that had knocked on the door was exiting the next door room with a worried look on his face. Outside the room, there was a whole array of medical equipment. I realised there was an emergency going on. I went around the corner and up the corridor to the communal area. I saw at the far end of this area my family with extremely worried looks on their faces. My mother came up to me and hugged me with relief. When they had arrived they had seen the nurse, who had gone to fetch me from my room. The next thing he must have done is make a routine check on the next room. The next thing my parents knew was that the nurse was rushing out from having been to find me and returned in haste with medics back to where my room was. I hadn't of course at this time appeared as I didn't realise they were waiting for me. They understandably assumed the worse and that the medics had been called because they thought I was in trouble. After a gap of a few minutes I finally emerged, to find them in a state of

David Stocks

total panic.

This brought home to me the reality of depression. It can kill. At this moment in time I am assuming the worse that the man in the next room has died, as the police would have left by now if not. I also heard the words 'suspicious circumstances,' that has led me to believe that he has taken his own life and not died of natural causes. I don't believe for a moment anyone in the hospital would have killed him and it is an all too frequent outcome of severe depression, someone finally ending it all. I am filled with deep sorrow for a lonely soul, now lost to the wonders of creation and the grief and suffering of all his family and friends. I know through my insights that the spark of creation will continue outside his earthly body and he will be an angel manifested on another astral plane. But no one's time should be cut short in this domain. It may be that the man was saved, I can only hope so.

I am only here now, typing this, because Jules has kept a constant vigil on me and at times has literally had to beg me from killing myself. I now understand the full reality of it and it is not pleasant. I can only give hope to people who have trodden this dark path of depression. There *is* light at the end of the tunnel, there *is* hope, life *is* worth living. Here is hope for the future:

You are unique, the whole of creation is your construct, and you were given life to interact with

The Celtic Holy Grail Quest

this creation. Don't waste it. The whole universe is your plaything.

No matter where you are, what situation you are in, however bad things may seem, believe in yourself. Look to fellow suffers, in here lies empathy and if you touch on this you will see real beauty. For you have travelled a dark path; now realise there is light.

One lesson I have learned is that you must not dwell on the past or worry about the future, as everyone has unique potential. Go with the flow, live for the present, fully emerge yourself in the present, get active, learn a new skill. If you commit yourself wholeheartedly to the present, you will know nothing but joy from now on.

In this desperate hour I now caught a glimpse of the Holy Grail.

A secret of the Grail is to be found in this poem; oh seekers of the Grail, interpret it as you will. Decipher what lies within.

> Step through the looking glass,
> Be careful who you meet,
> Let all the clocks stop,
> Who is it you seek?
>
> The corporeal is now ethereal,
> Surrounded by false noise,
> Cocooned from distraction,

David Stocks

On this inner voyage.

Floating in a cosmic soup,
Bathing in a starry bowl,
Galaxies spiral down,
Into a black hole.

Unfold the wings of creation,
Dew drops in the mind's vessel,
From which everything begins,
A sacred Celtic spell.

To get to this point, I have followed the Grail quest. In one version of the quest, Perceval meets the Fisher King at a lake, who appears as a fisherman. Perceval asks the fisherman how to ford a river that blocks his route. The Fisher King replies that there is no crossing nearby, but to please accept his hospitality and take a rest. His direction to his home is: go down the road, bear left, and cross the drawbridge. Perceval, who had been given these instructions before and found an enchanted castle, had forgotten to ask the question 'Whom does the grail serve?' He now realises that this is the Fisher King and poses the question.

I have followed these directions of the Fisher King; gone down the road (embarked on the quest within myself), followed my intuition and thought outside of the box (bear left), then gone deeper into my inner world (crossed the drawbridge), at the end of which lies my Grail.

The Celtic Holy Grail Quest

To reach the Grail I must pose the Fisher King a question. But who is the Fisher King? When I look for the Fisher King, I see only myself. For I realise that the Fisher King's land that has been made barren, is the wasteland of my mind. The Fisher King will be something different in everybody, but if you look carefully enough, the Fisher King will be there. So I pose the question:-
'Whom does the Grail serve?'

Looking into my heart, I now see the answer to that question.

Forgiveness.

We must first of all learn to forgive ourselves, or we can never be at one with creation and we must also learn to forgive all others. By the process of forgiving, all internal and external conflicts will end and the Fisher King can be healed.

The answer had been revealed to me on my quest, when I read the book 'The Art of Happiness' by the Dalai Lama. It is a core Buddhist value and it is truly the source of happiness. I had glimpsed this truth on my journey through the Celtic labyrinth that formed my quest for the Grail. I must have been close to the truth, but the labyrinth led me away again. The journey has ended back at the start of the labyrinth and I have achieved understanding. It is said, to find the Grail you must first be purified by pain and suffering. We must

David Stocks

lose ourselves in order to find ourselves, but we are frightened to let go. Once we are humbled, exhausted, or have even given up, we may be ready to stumble into the Grail chapel. My chapel is here in the Dorothy Pattison hospital.

Through forgiveness, we gain empathy with all other beings and can share love and an appreciation of creation.

I will leave you with a poem I wrote when I arrived at this hospital as it is an experience that transformed me and made me realise what fantastic company I am in. If you are depressed, take heart in it, for it applies to every single one of you. I still need time to recuperate and if you are depressed make sure you give yourself that time, but I feel healed now and am looking forward to the rest of my life.

Unity

Compatriots of despair,
Gather together in hope,
For companionship brings light,
Dark shadows cast aside.

Fellows despondent no more,
Stand united and proud,
There is no greater beauty on earth,
Than what we share inside.

The Celtic Holy Grail Quest

My quest has not finished yet, for although I have encountered the Fisher King and asked 'Whom does the Grail serve?' I have received an answer from within; there is still a lot more Grail legend to be uncovered.

www.ingramcontent.com/pod-product-compliance
Lightning Source LLC
Chambersburg PA
CBHW021831220426
43663CB00005B/205